I.V. Therapy Demystified

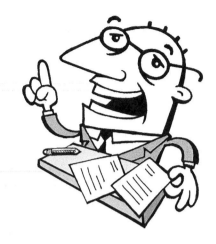

I.V. Therapy Demystified

Kerry H. Cheever, PhD, RN
Professor and Chairperson
St. Luke's Hospital School of Nursing
Moravian College
Assistant Vice President for Nursing
St. Luke's Hospital and Health Network
Bethlehem, Pennsylvania

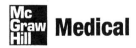

New York   Chicago   San Francisco   Lisbon   London
Madrid   Mexico City   Milan   New Delhi   San Juan
Seoul   Singapore   Sydney   Toronto

I.V. Therapy Demystified

3 4 5 6 7 8 9 0   QDB/QDB   12

ISBN   978-0-07-149678-0
MHID   0-07-149678-5

This book was set in Times Roman by International Typesetting and Composition.
The editors were Quincy McDonald and Robert Pancotti.
The production supervisor was Catherine Saggese.
Project management was provided by Preeti Longia Sinha, International Typesetting and Composition.
Cover design art directed by Margaret Webster-Shapiro.
The cover designer was Lance Lekander.
Quad/Graphics is the printer and binder.

This book is printed on acid-free paper.

Library of Congress Cataloging-in-Publication Data

Cheever, Kerry H.
  I.V. therapy demystified / Kerry H. Cheever.
      p. ; cm.
  Includes bibliographical references and index.
  ISBN-13: 978-0-07-149678-0 (pbk. : alk. paper)
  ISBN-10: 0-07-149678-5
  1. Intravenous therapy. 2. Nursing. I. Title. II. Title: IV therapy demystified.
[DNLM: 1. Infusions, Intravenous—nursing. WB 354 C527i 2008]
RM170.C464 2008
615.8'55—dc22

2007034873

To my parents, Thomas G. Hickey and Jane A. Rowan Hickey.
Dad—Thanks for paying my college tuition bills.
Mom—Thanks for not letting me give up on long division when I was in third grade.

CONTENTS

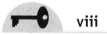

Contents

INTRODUCTION

Most patients admitted to hospitals today receive intravenous (I.V.) therapy. Indeed, it is estimated that over 90 percent of all hospitalized patients in the United States receive some form of I.V. therapy. Common indications for I.V. therapy include achieving or maintaining fluid and electrolyte balance, replacing or supplementing needed blood components, providing nutrients, and administering medications.

Nonclinicians may assume that clinicians are well versed in the initiation and maintenance of I.V. therapy simply because its use is so widespread. As a nurse educator with almost 20 years of teaching experience, I believe that this is not necessarily true, particularly among novice clinicians. Rather, I find that both novice nurses and student nurses frequently are mystified by basic principles that govern I.V. therapy initiation and maintenance. Even fairly simple concepts that could be readily understood if introduced properly seem foreign to both novices and students. For instance, in the not-so-distant past, when I supervised groups of junior- and senior-level nursing students enrolled in clinical medical/surgical practicum experiences, we would end our clinical practice days with the sacrosanct *postconferences,* which are informal seminar discussions typically mandated in most nursing curricula. During the course of any given term, I made certain that at least one postconference was devoted to basic principles of I.V. solutions. It was a sobering experience to find that most students could not readily identify the differences between crystalloid and colloid solutions, and few even understood differences among types of blood components and their indications beyond the use of packed red blood cells.

Although these nursing students whom I supervised in clinical practice had numerous resources on I.V. therapy at their disposal, those resources tended to be scattered among multiple sources. For instance, "cookbook" information on recommended steps to initiate and maintain I.V. therapy could be found in these students' "fundamentals" textbook, whereas information on blood component therapy typically was found in the "medical/surgical" textbook, and information on I.V. medications could be found in the "pharmacology" or "drug guide" textbooks.

There are indeed some excellent comprehensive textbooks on I.V. therapy that are available for purchase and review. However, those textbooks are almost too all-inclusive for the nursing student or the novice nurse to digest. A book that clearly identifies basic tenets that guide I.V. therapy for novice nurses and student nurses isn't available, and most novices learn these principles by the old and somewhat scary "OJT" (i.e., on-the-job training) method, which is, at best, spotty!

The intent behind the writing and publication of this book is to fill that gap and to provide a readily understandable basic resource on I.V. therapy for student and novice nurses. Most of the content contained in these chapters is derived from content that I delivered over a series of postconferences held with my former medical/surgical nursing students. These students generally found the content helpful, and many continued to stay in touch with me for years after graduation and affirmed that I gave them essential content that they continued to apply to their everyday practice.

This book is not a comprehensive treatise on I.V. therapy. For instance, there is no chapter devoted to chemotherapeutic agents. Only nurses who are well versed beyond the level of novice should be delivering I.V. chemotherapeutic agents. This book is written strictly for novices and students so that they may better understand basic principles of I.V. therapy.

A LOOK INSIDE

Each chapter in this book contains basic information that may help novice and student nurses to deliver I.V. therapy more competently to their patients in their daily practices. Each chapter begins with a set of novice-level Learning Objectives that outline the important concepts the reader should focus on learning. Some important concepts are immediately reinforced through fill-in-the-blank "Speed Bumps." Each chapter is written so that the concepts are easy to comprehend. Each chapter is also written succinctly so that busy students and novices may readily digest the concepts. Several multiple-choice questions are included at the end of each chapter so that readers may try to confirm that they can synthesize key content of the chapter. These multiple-choice items are written to mimic nursing board examination (i.e., NCLEX-RN) items and constitute another useful feature that may help nursing students better prepare to take that important examination successfully.

Chapter 1: Introduction to Intravenous Therapy

Chapter 1 "sets the stage" for the remainder of the book: It is the introductory chapter to I.V. therapy. Intravenous therapy is identified as a type of infusion therapy. The roles and responsibilities of nurses who care for patients receiving I.V. therapy are identified, as are the competencies that nurses must possess to attain specialty certification in I.V. therapy. Indications for patients to receive I.V. therapy are identified. Although I.V. therapy is commonly indicated for today's hospitalized inpatients, it is a relatively new phenomenon. Therefore, the historical evolution of I.V. therapy is also discussed in this chapter.

Chapter 2: Fluids and Electrolytes

To be able to understand principles of I.V. therapy, nurses must understand basic principles of fluid and electrolyte balance. Therefore, this chapter is a primer of important basic concepts of fluids and electrolytes. Normal composition of fluids and electrolytes in the intracellular and extracellular compartments are identified. Physiologic mechanisms that maintain fluid and electrolyte balance are discussed. Properties that define isotonic, hypotonic, and hypertonic solutions are presented, as are properties of key important physiologic electrolytes, which include sodium, chloride, potassium, magnesium, calcium, and phosphorus. Intravenous therapy indications for treatment of disturbances of fluids and electrolytes are also described.

Chapter 3: Intravenous Therapy Delivery Systems

This chapter identifies typical I.V. delivery systems and contains several accompanying figures that display key features of I.V. delivery systems. The reader is introduced to I.V. therapy containers, infusion sets, administration sets, and pumps. Commonly used terms used in practice, including *spiking* and *priming*, are defined and their usages discussed. Finally, methods to manually calculate I.V. drip rates with a variety of administration sets are described, with several exemplar problems.

Chapter 4: Peripheral Intravenous Therapy

Chapter 4 is devoted exclusively to the peripheral route of I.V. therapy and clearly identifies indications for initiating and maintaining this route of infusion. Some chapters in this book tend to be more theoretical (e.g., Chapter 2), whereas others are practical "how to" chapters. Chapter 4 falls into the latter category. Steps that may be followed to initiate a peripheral I.V. line are included in this chapter.

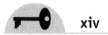

Peripheral venous access devices are compared and contrasted in terms of their design features and their preferred indications for usage. Methods that may help to provide stability to I.V. access devices are described. Steps for how to change an I.V. infusion set, change an I.V. access-site dressing, and discontinue an administration setup are all included in this chapter.

Chapter 5: Central Intravenous Therapy

This is another "how to" chapter. Whereas Chapter 4 targets the how-tos of peripheral I.V. therapy, Chapter 5 targets the key how-tos of central I.V. therapy. Indications for delivering I.V. therapy by the central route rather than the peripheral route are identified. Commonly used access devices to deliver central I.V. therapy are compared and contrasted in terms of their design features and their indications; they include peripherally inserted central catheters (PICCs), tunneled central venous catheters, percutaneous central venous catheters, and implanted ports. Adverse events associated with the use of these devices are also described. Steps for how to insert a PICC line and how to discontinue a PICC line or a nontunneled central access line are also described.

Chapter 6: Intravenous Therapy and the Nursing Process

The principles described in Chapter 6 are probably the most important in the book because they describe the applicability of the steps of the nursing process for nurses who care for patients who receive I.V. therapy. The interplay between actual and potential nursing diagnoses, nursing outcomes, and nursing interventions for patients receiving I.V. therapy are described in a user-friendly, generic format. The reader can readily tailor these guidelines individually when crafting care plans for patients receiving I.V. therapy.

Chapter 7: Crystalloid Solutions

This chapter targets crystalloid I.V. solutions exclusively and identifies characteristics of the composition of various types of crystalloid solutions, including those that are primarily sodium-based, those that are primarily dextrose-based, and those that contain a complex mixture of electrolytes. The chapter contains information that enables the reader to distinguish among isotonic, hypotonic, and hypertonic crystalloid solutions. The chapter also discusses physiologic responses that occur when crystalloid solutions are infused and indications for selection and maintenance of commonly prescribed crystalloid solutions.

Chapter 8: Colloid Solutions

Chapter 8 mirrors the format of Chapter 7 but targets colloid solutions rather than crystalloid solutions. Colloid solutions are compared and contrasted with crystalloid solutions. Characteristics of the composition of various types of colloids are described, including those that are nonsynthetic and those that are synthetic. The indications for the use of albumin, plasma protein fraction (PPF), Hespan, dextran, and gelatins are described, as are common adverse events associated with their use.

Chapter 9: Blood Component Therapy

Chapter 9 describes indications for commonly transfused blood components and their most commonly associated adverse events. This chapter contains both theoretical content and "how to" application pieces. Blood components described include whole blood, packed red blood cells (PRBCs), fresh-frozen plasma (FFP), platelets, immunoglobulins, and clotting factors (e.g., cryoprecipitate). Steps for how to ensure the safe delivery of blood component I.V. therapy are described.

Chapter 10: Parenteral Nutrition Therapy

Chapter 10 targets principles of parenteral I.V. therapy and has a format similar to that of Chapter 9 in that it contains both theoretical information and "how to" information. Indications for delivering nutrients parenterally are described, and common types of parenteral solutions are compared and contrasted, including total parenteral nutrition (TPN) solutions, total nutrient admixtures (TNAs), and fat emulsions. Continuous and cyclic methods of delivering parenteral nutrition are compared and contrasted, as are indications for using central versus peripheral access routes. There are many adverse events that may be associated with the delivery of parenteral I.V. therapy, and the most common of these are described. Steps for how to initiate, monitor, and discontinue parenteral I.V. therapy are each clearly described.

Chapter 11: Intravenous Pharmacologic Therapy

There are many resources to which student and novice nurses may refer for administering I.V. medications. There are textbooks devoted exclusively to this topic. In addition, most "drug guides" for nurses contain a plethora of information on I.V. medications under each individually listed agent, including mode of delivery, medication and solution compatibilities and incompatibilities, and recommended delivery intervals. This book certainly does not address all those minute details. What this book does provide is a succinct yet salient overview of

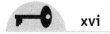
important practical concepts that the nurse must understand in order to deliver I.V. medications safely and effectively. In addition, the prototype drugs for the class of I.V. medications that are prescribed most commonly are listed in one convenient table that provides an overview of key administration guidelines and important incompatibilities.

Chapter 12: Intravenous Therapy and Infants and Children

Chapter 12 provides a concise overview of key differences between administering I.V. therapy to infants and children and administering to adults. The chapter compares and contrasts I.V. delivery systems, I.V. access devices, and I.V. solutions indicated for use in infants and children with those commonly used in adults. Basic competencies that the nurse must master to deliver I.V. therapy safely and effectively to infants and children are identified. Although this is an I.V. therapy book, this chapter identifies and briefly describes alternate infusion access sites that are used commonly in children and infants, including intraosseous sites and umbilical veins and arteries, respectively, so that student and novice nurses may glean a basic understanding of their indications.

Chapter 13: Intravenous Therapy and the Older Adult

Chapter 13 is formatted so that it mirrors Chapter 12. It is another chapter that targets a special population that may receive I.V. therapy, the older adult. Initiating and maintaining I.V. therapy in older adults can pose unique challenges. Age-related physiologic changes that dictate changes in selection and maintenance of I.V. access sites and selection and delivery of solutions are described. This chapter also identifies and briefly describes an alternate infusion delivery method that may be used in the older adult: hypodermoclysis.

Chapter 14: Intravenous Therapy within Community-Based Settings

The use of I.V. therapy as a therapeutic option has increased not only in the inpatient environment but also in the outpatient environment. It has become common that patients (i.e., clients) in community-based settings receive I.V. therapy. This chapter provides a brief overview of community-based settings where I.V. therapy may be delivered and identifies the role of the nurse in terms of ensuring safe and effective delivery of I.V. therapy within these settings. Community-based nurses spend much time and many resources teaching patients and families how to care for themselves safely and effectively. Thus the role of the nurse in teaching these patients and families how to deliver I.V. therapy safely and effectively and maintain vascular access sites is described.

Reference

1. Corrigan AM: History of intravenous therapy. In Hankins J, Lonsway RA, Hedrick, C, et al. (eds.): *Infusion Therapy in Clinical Practice*, 2nd ed. Philadelphia: Saunders, 2001.

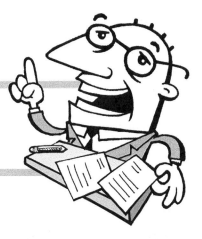

CHAPTER 1

Introduction to Intravenous Therapy

Learning Objectives

After completing this chapter, the learner will

1. Define *infusion therapy* and *intravenous (I.V.) therapy* and distinguish between them.

2. Describe the historical evolution of I.V. therapy.

3. Recognize the nurse's role and responsibility in ensuring safe and competent delivery of I.V. therapy.

4. Appreciate the basic requirements to attain specialty certification in infusion therapy.

5. List common indications for initiating I.V. therapy.

Key Terms

Infusion therapy
Parenteral
I.V. therapy

Therapy Defined

1 Intravenous (I.V.) therapy is sometimes more broadly referred to as *infusion therapy*. These terms are not exactly synonymous, however. **Infusion therapy** is defined as the parenteral infusion of fluids, electrolytes, blood components, nutrients, or medications to prevent or treat deficiencies or diseases. The term **parenteral** refers to a route of administration of a therapeutic agent, and the parenteral route of administration is any route other than one that involves the gastrointestinal tract (e.g., oral or rectal route) or a topical route (e.g., optic or dermal route). Infusion therapy may be dispensed by I.V., subcutaneous, intraosseous, or intrathecal routes of administration. **I.V. therapy** is a type of infusion therapy that is confined to administration of fluids, electrolytes, blood components, nutrients, or medications by the I.V. route.

SPEED BUMP

_____ *is defined as the parenteral infusion of fluids, electrolytes, blood components, nutrients, or medications to prevent or treat deficiencies or diseases.*

Historical Evolution of I.V. Therapy

2 Although a very common therapy today, I.V. therapy was used rarely as a treatment option until close to the middle of the twentieth century. The role of nurses in initiating and maintaining I.V. therapy, while unquestioned now, was not established until after the end of World War II.[1]

The first known attempts at establishing I.V. therapy occurred during the Renaissance with attempts to transfuse either animal blood to humans or presumably noncrossmatched blood from human to human. Not surprisingly, the results tended to be lethal. As a result, the practice of transfusing blood was banned in Europe for a considerable time following the demise of several test subjects, including a pope.[2]

In the 1830s, a lethal strain of cholera wracked much of Europe. This type of cholera was called "Russian cholera," for the supposed country of its origin, or "blue cholera," for the dusky cyanotic complexion of its victims. It was associated with severe diarrhea and dehydration. A 22-year-old Scottish physician, William Brooke O'Shaughnessy, hypothesized that the primary cause of death in persons who succumbed to blue cholera was a deficiency of fluids and electrolytes. He postulated that replacing these deficient fluids and electrolytes in a solution infused in the patients' veins could be effective and possibly lifesaving therapy. A physician colleague of Dr. O'Shaughnessy, Thomas Latta, was the first to implement this then-novel therapy with blue cholera patients, and he reported that although not all patients survived, the outcomes were nonetheless much improved. This new practice was ridiculed by most of Dr. O'Shaughnessy's and Dr. Latta's physician contemporaries, who were more inclined to practice traditional medical therapies, including blood letting with leaches and inducing emesis.[3,4] Nonetheless, this marked a sentinel event generally recognized in health science as the advent of I.V. therapy.

Toward the end of the nineteenth century, saline- and glucose-based I.V. solutions were used to treat the critically ill. Although the primitive I.V. delivery systems used during this period were designed to be reusable, a new understanding of the role of microbial organisms in the transmission of diseases meant that these systems were sterilized between patients. These delivery systems were cumbersome and difficult to use and maintain. For instance, these systems typically included steel-tipped I.V. needles that were taped in place once I.V. access was obtained. These I.V. access needles then were connected to tubing that led to open glass cylinders filled with solution and covered with sterile gauze.[2] Many complications were associated with this type of I.V. system that are difficult to appreciate today. For instance, it was difficult to maintain system asepsis, infiltration into the surrounding tissues occurred frequently after I.V. access was initiated, and maintaining prescribed solution administration rates required a great deal of vigilance and time. Because these delivery systems were primitive and fraught with difficulties, only the most moribund patients were prescribed I.V. therapy in the early decades of the twentieth century. As a result, the initiation and monitoring of I.V. therapy during this period of time were wholly within the domain of the physician and remained so for the next several decades.[1]

During the early twentieth century, medical science first appreciated the significance of antigen-antibody reactions, ABO blood types, and Rh factor compatibility, thus paving the way for effective and safe transfusion of blood and blood component products. Blood transfusion therapy made its greatest scientific strides during World War II, providing lifesaving treatment to young soldiers, seamen, airmen, and marines who suffered traumatic injuries.[2] On the heels of these advances, with the rise of the science of anesthesiology during the worldwide poliomyelitis pandemic, I.V. access sites began to be used more commonly as a quick and convenient route to administer a variety of medications. I.V. delivery systems became single-use disposable systems that were easier to initiate and use. Over-the-needle catheter I.V. access devices were designed that infiltrated less frequently than the needle-based I.V. access devices. I.V. delivery systems were designed as "closed systems" with secure tubing connections and quality-controlled drip regulators that led to closed bottles that contained sterile solution. Delivery of medications by syringe bolus methods (i.e., I.V. push), I.V. "piggyback" methods, and continuous I.V. infusions became easy to achieve and therefore more commonplace.

With the introduction of higher-quality closed delivery systems, physicians began to prescribe I.V. therapy more commonly to patients who were not necessarily moribund. As more and more physiologically stable patients received I.V. therapy, physicians began to delegate the responsibility to monitor patients receiving I.V. therapy to nurses. By the latter half of the twentieth century, state medical boards consented that initiation of peripheral I.V. access was a procedure that could be shared with professional nurses.[1]

Until the 1960s, the complement of nutrients present in any I.V. solution was not sufficient to meet daily caloric and other nutritional requirements. It was a common observation that patients with critical illnesses and patients with debilitating chronic illnesses were unable to consume sufficient nutrients orally and lost lean muscle mass. Loss of lean muscle mass, in turn, resulted in susceptibility to infections and poor wound healing.[5] Total parenteral nutrition (TPN) I.V. solutions were introduced in the late 1960s to provide a source of essential nutrients and calories to these patients.[2]

I.V. Therapy Today

I.V. therapy is a very commonplace therapeutic treatment today. Indeed, it is estimated that over 90 percent of all hospitalized inpatients in the United States are recipients of I.V. therapy.[2] Moreover, I.V. therapies are not restricted to the inpatient hospital environment. I.V. therapies are prescribed and used commonly in same-day surgery centers, long-term care facilities, outpatient clinics, and home health settings. **3** The nurse is typically the professional who is responsible for maintaining, monitoring, and evaluating the effectiveness of I.V. therapy. The nurse is frequently also responsible for gaining I.V. access and initiating infusions. In many nursing practice settings, a great deal of the nurse's time and professional responsibility revolve around competent delivery of I.V. therapy. Therefore, it is vitally important that today's nurses understand at least the basic principles of I.V. therapy. The nurse responsible for ensuring safe and effective I.V. therapy must be capable of the following:

- Understanding the basic principles of fluid and electrolyte balance
- Selecting and maintaining appropriate I.V. delivery systems
- Recognizing common principles that guide the initiation and maintenance of peripheral and central I.V. access sites
- Formulating common nursing diagnoses, identifying common nursing outcomes, and ensuring appropriate nursing interventions for patients receiving I.V. therapy
- Differentiating common crystalloid solutions, colloidal solutions, blood component products, and parenteral nutritional therapy solutions in terms of indications for their use and key adverse events associated with their use
- Identifying principles that guide competent and safe administration of medications via the I.V. route of delivery
- Recognizing basic principles that guide competent and safe administration of I.V. therapy in special populations, including pediatric and gerontologic populations, as well as populations in community-based settings

This book provides a broad overview of these basic principles of I.V. therapy that can help guide the nurse in many practice settings. Nurses who wish to master advanced principles of I.V. therapy are encouraged to familiarize themselves with guidelines for I.V. therapy promulgated by the Infusion Nurses Society.[6] Infusion nursing is considered a specialized area of clinical practice. **4** Nurses who choose to hone advanced skills within this practice area may be eligible to take the Certified Registered Nurse Infusion (CRNI) certification examination that is developed and administered by the Infusion Nurses Certification Corporation (INCC), a subsidiary of the Infusion Nurses Society. In order to be eligible to take this examination, a registered nurse must demonstrate active licensure and at least 1600 hours of clinical practice in infusion therapy within the 2 years that precede taking the examination.[7]

Indications for I.V. Therapy

5 Indications for I.V. therapy include achieving or maintaining fluid and electrolyte balance, replacing or supplementing needed blood components, providing nutrients, and administering medications.

FLUID AND ELECTROLYTE BALANCE

Dehydration is a common indication for I.V. therapy. When patients lose body fluids in excess of fluid intake, not only may dehydration occur, but key electrolytes that serve to maintain homeostasis and serum osmolality also may become disrupted. Replacing fluids in patients who are dehydrated, therefore, is not a matter of merely replacing lost vascular volume. Not only must fluids be restored to the vasculature, but electrolyte levels also must be assessed and possibly treated as well.

Many times patients are given I.V. fluids to prevent a loss of fluids or electrolytes. For instance, the vast majority of surgical patients have I.V. fluids administered intraoperatively to maintain fluid balance. Likewise, during the postoperative period, when patients are not able to take oral fluids (i.e., they are NPO), I.V. fluids are administered to preserve fluid balance. Chapter 2 provides an overview of the role of I.V. therapy in preserving fluid and electrolyte balance.

BLOOD COMPONENT THERAPY

The earliest recorded efforts to commence I.V. therapy revolved around attempts to administer blood component products. Although these efforts were not effective for several centuries, this changed with the recognition of ABO blood typing and Rh factors. Once type and crossmatching of blood component products became readily available, the use of blood component products became commonplace, first with the transfusion of plasma, followed closely by the transfusion of other blood component products.[2] It is now commonplace therapy to transfuse packed red blood cells, fresh-frozen plasma, platelets, and clotting factors depending on their indications and demonstrated therapeutic effectiveness. For the most part, these transfusions are administered when a patient begins to exhibit clinical manifestations of a deficiency of the given blood component product. Chapter 9 provides a more comprehensive discussion of indications for transfusion of various blood component products.

SPEED BUMP

Common blood components that may be transfused include _____,
fresh-frozen plasma, platelets, and clotting factors.

PARENTERAL NUTRITION

Parenteral nutrition is a relatively new indication for I.V. therapy. Parenteral nutrition was not considered possible without causing serious and potentially lethal adverse effects until well into the 1960s.[2] Parenteral nutrition now is a safe and therapeutic treatment option for many patients. There are now a host of indications for parenteral therapy, and parenteral nutrient solution composition is determined individually to meet each patient's nutritional needs. In general, parenteral solutions tend to include nutrients that include electrolytes, dextrose, amino acids, vitamins, and various trace elements. These solutions are referred to as *total parenteral nutrition* (TPN). Most patients receiving TPN also require supplemental intravenous fat emulsions (IVFEs) to provide essential fats. There are also solutions referred to as *total nutrient admixture* (TNA) solutions that provide a nutrient mix that includes electrolytes, dextrose, amino acids, vitamins, trace elements, and fats. The concentration of nutrients in these solutions, including TPN solutions, IVFEs, and TNA solutions, is determined in part by the choice of I.V. delivery route. In general, the solutions are less concentrated when they are delivered by a peripheral I.V. route and are more concentrated when delivered by a central I.V. route. Chapter 10 provides a more complete overview of types of TPN, IVFEs, and TNA solutions and delivery routes.

Although TPN is an effective method to deliver nutrients to patients who cannot take nutrients orally, it is generally considered an inferior route of feeding to the enteral route.[5]

MEDICATION THERAPY

The last common indication for I.V. therapy is to ensure the effective delivery of pharmacologic agents. Some patients require continuous I.V. infusions of medications such as vasopressors (e.g., dopamine [Intropin] and norepinephrine [Levophed]). Others may require intermittent infusions of medications in I.V. solutions that can be "piggybacked" into their main I.V. lines, such as antibiotics (e.g., cefazolin [Ancef]). Some patients may need bolus doses of medications on an intermittent or as-needed basis, such as diuretic agents (e.g., furosemide [Lasix]). In some instances, patients with unstable physiologic status may have an I.V. access site set up "just in case" so that medications may be administered rapidly if there is an emergent or urgent indication (e.g., amiodarone [Cordarone] and epinephrine). In other instances, patients may have a chronic illness and require intermittent infusions of medications, and placing an I.V. access site into these patients that may be capped prevents their undergoing the trauma of repeated venipuncture to gain I.V. access. Chapter 11 provides a more complete overview of indications for I.V. pharmacologic therapy.

Summary

I.V. therapy is not a new therapeutic option to treat patients with a potential or actual deficiency in fluid and electrolytes, blood components, or nutrients or in need of medications. However, technological and scientific advancements over the course of the past few decades have resulted in a marked increase in the use of I.V. therapy. Most hospital inpatients and many patients in ambulatory and outpatient settings are prescribed I.V. therapy. There are a multitude of I.V. delivery systems, access sites, and solutions that the competent nurse must be comfortable using to deliver safe and effective care of patients receiving I.V. therapy.

Quiz

1. The parenteral route of administration includes which of the following routes:
    (a) Intravenous
    (b) Oral
    (c) Rectal
    (d) Optic

2. Infusion therapy includes *all but which* of the following routes of infusion?
    (a) Intravenous
    (b) Subcutaneous
    (c) Alimentary
    (d) Intrathecal

3. The professional organization that is responsible for developing and administering the Certified Registered Nurse Infusion (CRNI) examination is the
    (a) American Nurses Association.
    (b) Infusion Nurses Society.
    (c) Infusion Nurses Certification Corporation.
    (d) American Nurses Credentialing Center.

4. Common indications for I.V. therapy include
    (a) treating fatigue.
    (b) preventing diarrhea.
    (c) treating dehydration.
    (d) treating gastroenteritis.

5. Administering blood component products became more successful and hence more commonplace with the discovery of
    (a) ABO blood types.
    (b) blood product–compatible solutions.
    (c) specialized blood component product delivery systems.
    (d) platelet antigen-antibody crossmatching methods.

6. Administration of I.V. medications may be achieved by *all but which* of the following methods?
    (a) Continuous drip
    (b) Gastric infusion
    (c) Intermittent drip
    (d) "Piggyback" infusion

CHAPTER 2

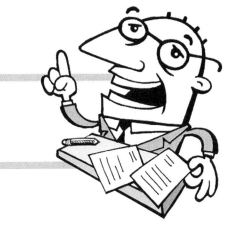

Fluids and Electrolytes

Learning Objectives

After completing this chapter, the learner will

1. Compare and contrast the normal composition of fluid and electrolytes in the intracellular fluid compartment with the extracellular fluid compartment.

2. Identify common passive transport, active transport, and physiologic homeostatic mechanisms that maintain fluid and electrolyte balance.

3. Describe isotonic, hypotonic, and hypertonic solutions.

4. Explain the role of key electrolytes, including sodium, chloride, potassium, magnesium, calcium, and phosphorus, in maintaining cellular and systemic function.

5. Recognize common causes and clinical manifestations of disturbances in sodium, chloride, potassium, magnesium, calcium, and phosphorus balance.

6. Describe common intravenous therapies indicated to treat disturbances in sodium, chloride, potassium, magnesium, calcium, and phosphorus balance.

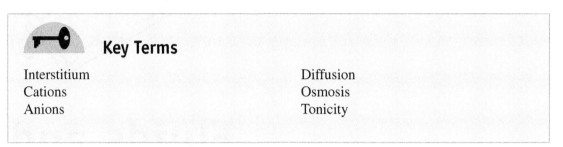

Key Terms

Interstitium	Diffusion
Cations	Osmosis
Anions	Tonicity

The human body is composed primarily of various fluids and electrolytes. Whenever there is some type of disruption in fluid balance or a disturbance in the normal levels of electrolytes, many different treatments and therapies may be indicated. Intravenous (I.V.) therapies are used quite commonly as one means to correct fluid and electrolyte abnormalities.

Body Fluids

Water comprises approximately 60 percent of total body weight in a normal-sized, healthy adult male. In general, fat contains less water than muscle. Therefore, people who are overweight have a lesser proportion of water that comprises their body weight. Similarly, women, children, and the elderly all tend to have less muscle mass than healthy adult men, and therefore, their bodies proportionately have less water. Those people with less water weight are susceptible to dehydration more quickly when stressed or ill because they have less reserve fluid.[8]

Daily fluid intake and output are approximately equivalent in healthy people. The average adult drinks 2–2.5 L of fluid daily, and normal digestion of foods and metabolism of their nutrients result in an intake of an additional 200–300 mL of water. The kidneys excrete 1.5–2 L of fluid (as urine) daily, approximately 300 mL of fluid is lost through bowel movements, and approximately 600 mL is lost via the skin and respiratory tract on a daily basis.[9]

Fluid Compartments

Body tissues and individual cells are bathed continuously in a *milieu interieur,*[10] or internal environment, of fluids that are composed primarily of water, electrolytes, molecular nutrients, macromolecules, and gases. This internal environment exists in three distinct spaces that include the intracellular, interstitial, and intravascular compartments, which are displayed in Fig. 2-1. The fluids in each of these compartments characteristically differ from each other in composition.

INTRACELLULAR FLUID

1 Approximately two-thirds of all bodily fluids reside within the body's cells. The intracellular fluid (ICF) compartment is separated from the extracellular fluid (ECF) compartment by the cell membrane. The fluid within the cell is a tad bit more acidic than the fluid in the external environment. The cell membrane is porous, or semipermeable, so that water may pass easily through either side of this membrane.

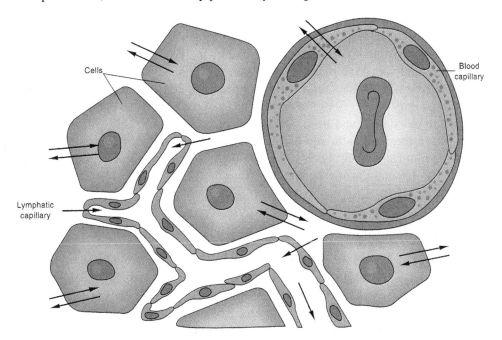

Figure 2-1   Body water moves between the intracellular fluid (ICF) compartment and the extracellular fluid (ECF) compartment, which includes the interstitial and intravascular spaces. (Reprinted with permission from Nowak TJ, Handford AG: *Essentials of Pathophysiology: Concepts and Applications for Health Care Professionals*, 2nd ed. Boston: WCB/McGraw-Hill, 1999:406.)

However, most electrolytes, nutrients, and molecules cannot pass readily through the cell membrane but may enter or exit selectively through active transport mechanisms that include port systems and pump systems. For instance, most of the body's potassium at any point in time resides within body cells, whereas most of the body's sodium at any point in time lies outside the cells' interior environment. This is so because the sodium–potassium pump ensures that most of the sodium is pumped out of the cell, whereas most of the potassium is pumped into the cell.[8]

EXTRACELLULAR FLUID

The extracellular fluid (ECF) compartment includes any body fluid that does not exist within the body cells. This fluid accounts for one-third of all body fluid. ECF compartments are further subdivided into interstitial fluid and intravascular fluid compartments.

Interstitium

The **interstitium**, otherwise referred to as the *interstitial space* or the *third space,* contains fluid that bathes the exterior of body cells but does not lie within a vascular compartment. Vascular compartments include major blood vessels such as arteries and veins and microvasculature such as distal capillaries. The fluid in the interstitium resembles fluid within the vascular compartment except that in a normal, healthy state it does not contain any red blood cells or platelets and very few white blood cells and little albumin. There is a considerable volume of body fluid that resides within the interstitium because it accounts for 80 percent of ECF volume.[9] Fluid and electrolytes may shift into and out of the interstitium from the ICF across the cellular membrane and from the vasculature across the capillary membrane.

Intravascular

Blood is the fluid that is contained within the intravascular compartment. In a normal-sized, healthy adult, blood is composed of 40 percent cells, including red blood cells (i.e., erythrocytes), white blood cells (i.e., leukocytes), and platelets (i.e., thrombocytes). The remaining 60 percent balance of blood that is not composed of cells is called *plasma* and contains water, electrolytes, and various macromolecules, including fibrinogen, globulins, and albumin. Plasma accounts for only 20 percent of all the ECF. Albumin is the macromolecule that is primarily responsible for maintaining colloidal osmotic pressure (COP). The COP must be maintained within a certain discrete range so that normal volumes of plasma can be maintained within the vascular compartment and will not diffuse into the interstitium.[8]

Electrolytes

Simply stated, *electrolytes* are chemical ions that are important in maintaining organic function. The concentration of electrolytes is measured in milliequivalents per liter of fluid (i.e., mEq/L). Electrolytes carry an electrical-like charge, called an *ionic charge,* that may be either positive or negative. In general, positively and negatively charged ions may attract each other, bond, and form salts. For instance, when sodium (i.e., Na^+) meets chloride (i.e., Cl^-), they form sodium chloride (i.e., NaCl), otherwise known as *table salt.* On the other hand, two positively charged ions that meet will repel each other, as will two negatively charged ions.

CATIONS

Electrolytes in body fluids that are positively charged are called **cations**. The most common cations include sodium (i.e., Na^+), potassium (i.e., K^+), calcium (i.e., Ca^{2+}), and magnesium (i.e., Mg^{2+}). As noted previously, sodium is the major extracellular electrolyte, whereas potassium is the major intracellular electrolyte.

ANIONS

Body fluid electrolytes that are negatively charged are called **anions**. The most common anions include chloride (i.e., Cl^-), bicarbonate (i.e., HCO_3^-), and phosphate (i.e., PO_4^{3-}). Chloride and bicarbonate are the major extracellular anions, and phosphate is the main intracellular anion.

Mechanisms that Maintain Fluid and Electrolyte Balance

2 A host of mechanisms helps to maintain fluid and electrolyte balance in the body and include passive transport mechanisms, active transport mechanisms, and physiologic homeostatic mechanisms, and these are discussed in the following sections.

PASSIVE TRANSPORT

Passive transport mechanisms do not require the body to expend any energy in the form of adenosine triphosphate (ATP) for the mechanism to occur.

Diffusion

Diffusion is defined as the movement of particles from an area of greater concentration to an area of lesser concentration until equilibrium occurs.

Osmosis

Osmosis is defined as the movement of water across a semipermeable membrane from an area of lesser concentration of solute (e.g., more dilute solution) to an area of greater solute concentration (e.g., less dilute solution) until equilibrium occurs. The pressure that is generated from this movement is referred to as *osmotic pressure.*

ACTIVE TRANSPORT

Active transport mechanisms operate in opposition to passive transport mechanisms in that they do require energy expenditure in the form of ATP to occur. The objective of these mechanisms tends to revolve around maintaining the distinct features of each fluid compartment. The intracellular environment has a much different composition of electrolytes than the extracellular environment, as displayed in Table 2-1, and this difference is maintained by active transport mechanisms. An example of an active transport mechanism is the sodium–potassium pump, which serves to pump sodium out of the cell and keep potassium within the cell. Disruption in this pump can result in two lethal complications. First of all, serum hyperkalemia may occur, which can result in lethal cardiac dysrhythmias. Second, the sodium level within the cell will increase, and water will passively follow into the cell via osmosis, resulting in cell swelling and eventual cellular rupture.[8]

Table 2-1   Composition of Electrolytes in Intravascular Extracellular Fluid (ECF) and Intracellular Fluid (ICF)

Electrolyte	Intravascular ECF	ICF
Sodium	140 mEq/L	10 mEq/L
Potassium	4 mEq/L	150 mEq/L
Chloride	102 mEq/L	3 mEq/L
Magnesium	2.5 mEq/L	40 mEq/L
Calcium	5 mEq/L	<1 mEq/L
Phosphate	2 mEq/L	100 mEq/L

PHYSIOLOGIC MECHANISMS

There are several physiologic mechanisms that serve to maintain fluid and electrolyte homeostasis. Some of these mechanisms require the expenditure of energy, and others do not. Whenever there is a disruption in any of these mechanisms, whether it is because of an acute or chronic illness, the consequence is that fluid and electrolyte balance is disrupted.

Capillary–Interstitium Fluid Exchange

Fluid moves continuously between the capillary space and the interstitial space. This is possible because capillary filtration pressure pushes fluid from the capillary to the interstitium, whereas capillary COP pushes fluid back into the capillary. In addition to these capillary-induced mechanisms, fluid pressure within the interstitium opposes capillary filtration pressure, and interstitial COP pulls fluid into the interstitial space. In essence, normal composition of solutes within the capillary and interstitial spaces is necessary to ensure that these forces remain in equilibrium. The most common cause of disequilibrium between these forces is a deficiency of albumin in the vascular space.

Albumin

Albumin and the globulins and fibrinogen are the major proteins found in plasma and hence are collectively referred to as the *plasma proteins.* Albumin is the main determinant of COP. Indeed, over 75 percent of COP is maintained by albumin.[11] Therefore, serum albumin levels must be at least at the lower end of normal for normal COP to be maintained. In general, a normal serum albumin level in adults is 3.5–5.0 mg/dL and for children is 4.0–5.9 mg/dL.[11] If serum albumin levels are lower than normal, a condition referred to as *hypoalbuminemia,* then capillary COP cannot be maintained, and fluid seeps into the interstitium. This may result in fluid retention in the tissues and weight gain, although this gain in weight reflects gain in fluid rather than a gain in muscle mass or fat stores.

Starvation and lack of appropriate nutrients commonly cause hypoalbuminemia. In addition, acute stress is a common cause. During times of acute stress, whether the stressor is a disease or an injury, the liver manufactures increased amounts of acute-phase reactant proteins, including complement and gamma globulins, in order to mount a defense against the threat of the stressor. As a result, the liver may not be able to continue to manufacture sufficient quantities of albumin. This phenomenon is referred to as *hepatic reprioritization* and partially explains why critically ill patients are almost always hypoalbuminemic and at risk for fluid retention in the interstitial space.[5] Indeed, some critically ill patients may have widespread systemic edema to the extent that they exhibit what is referred to as a *kwashiorkor* appearance.[5]

Because albumin plays such a key role in maintaining COP, it is used frequently as a colloid I.V. therapy to treat patients who are critically ill or who have a significant nutritional deficit, often with mixed results. Please refer to Chapter 8 for a further discussion of albumin I.V. therapy.

Thirst Center

The thirst center, which is located in the hypothalamus, regulates fluid balance. Specialized neurons referred to as *osmoreceptors* sense serum osmolality, and when it increases, reflecting dehydration, thirst is stimulated. The thirst center also can be triggered indirectly by baroreceptors that are located in large vessels such as the aortic arch and the carotids. These baroreceptors are sensitive to pressure or stretch and are triggered by a decrease in blood volume.[8]

Kidneys

The renal tubules in the kidneys can selectively reabsorb or diurese water and electrolytes as needed to maintain fluid volume balance. The renal tubules respond to several different mechanisms. First of all, in the presence of low oxygen tension that results from either a low hemoglobin level or a decrease in blood volume, the juxtaglomerular cells within the kidneys produce the hormone renin. Renin has the effect of converting a relatively inert plasma protein called *angiotensinogen* to angiotensin I. When angiotensin I enters the pulmonary vascular circuit, it meets angiotensin-converting enzyme, which converts it to angiotensin II. Angiotensin II causes systemic vasoconstriction, resulting in an increase in systemic arterial blood pressure, and it influences the renal tubules so that sodium and water are reabsorbed. The effects of angiotensin II are relatively short-lived; however, it also stimulates the adrenals to release aldosterone. Aldosterone has similar effects to angiotensin II, including a systemic increase in blood pressure through its vasoconstrictive effects. Moreover, it also encourages the renal tubules to reabsorb more sodium and water. Its effects are longer-lived than those of angiotensin II.[8]

Antidiuretic Hormone

Antidiuretic hormone (ADH) affects the renal tubules directly so that increased reabsorption of water occurs. ADH is a hormone that is stored and released by the posterior portion of the pituitary gland, otherwise called the *neurohypophysis,* when it is stimulated by the thirst center in the hypothalamus. As noted previously, the thirst center responds to input from osmoreceptors, which are particularly receptive to subtle changes in serum osmolality and to input from vascular baroreceptors, which, in turn, are receptive to acute changes in blood volume.[8]

Fluid Tonicity

3 The **tonicity** of a fluid is a term that refers to the osmolality of a fluid specimen. Osmolality is a measure of osmotically active particles in a given solution for a unit of mass. The majority of these osmotically active particles are electrolytes. Specifically, tonicity refers to the osmolality of a given fluid as compared with the osmolality of the ICF of a cell that lies within a pool of that fluid. The effects of ECF tonicity on cells is displayed in Fig. 2-2 and is discussed in the following sections.

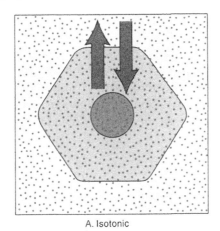

A. Isotonic

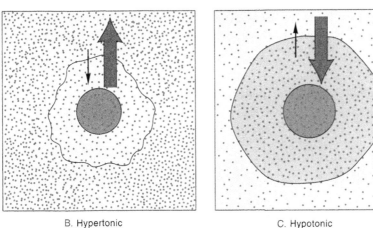

B. Hypertonic   C. Hypotonic

Figure 2-2 Note the effects of tonicity of solutions on cells. *A.* Cells placed in isotonic solutions maintain homeostasis. *B.* Cells placed in hypertonic solutions tend to lose intracellular fluid and shrink. *C.* Cells paced in hypotonic solutions tend to gain too much intracellular fluid and swell. (Reprinted with permission from Nowak TJ, Handford AG: *Essentials of Pathophysiology: Concepts and Applications for Health Care Professionals,* 2nd ed. Boston: WCB/McGraw-Hill, 1999:409.)

ISOTONIC

Isotonic fluids tend to have the same osmolality as plasma and therefore have approximately the same concentration of osmotically active particles in solution as ICF. Isotonic fluids have an approximate total electrolyte content of 310 mEq/L.[12] Therefore, a cell placed in a pool of isotonic fluid would neither swell nor shrink. An example of an isotonic solution is 0.9% normal saline (called *normal saline* or simply *saline*).

HYPOTONIC

Hypotonic fluids have a *lesser* concentration of osmotically active particles than ICF. The total electrolyte content of hypotonic fluids is less than 250 mEq/L.[12] Thus a cell placed in a pool of hypotonic solution would swell because water would move into the cell by osmosis. Some examples of hypotonic solutions include 0.45% saline (called *half-normal saline* or *½NS*) and water.

HYPERTONIC

Hypertonic solutions have a *greater* concentration of osmotically active particles than does plasma and can include solutions such as 5% dextrose in 0.9% normal saline (called D_5 *in normal saline* or D_5NS) and 25% mannitol. Electrolyte content of these fluids is at least 375 mEq/L.[12] A cell placed in a pool of hypertonic solution would shrink because water would exit the cell membrane via osmosis.

SPEED BUMP

Tonicity of a fluid refers to the concentration of particles, primarily _____, in the fluid.

Sodium Balance

4 Normal serum sodium levels range between 135 and 145 mEq/L. As the major serum cation, sodium plays a large role in maintaining serum osmolality and tonicity. It also is important in maintaining transport of glucose and insulin across the cell membrane and in facilitating the transmission of neuromuscular impulses.

HYPONATREMIA

5 A serum sodium level of less than 135 mEq/L defines *hyponatremia.* Common causes and clinical manifestations of hyponatremia are displayed in Table 2-2. Hyponatremia can be classified as hypervolemic, hypovolemic, and isovolemic.[13] Hypervolemic hyponatremia may result from chronic retention of fluid, caused by diseases such as heart failure and resulting in a proportionate decrease of sodium in the intravascular space. Hypovolemic hyponatremia generally results when fluid is lost acutely, and sodium loss proportionately exceeds the amount of fluid lost. Excessive vomiting and excessive sweating are examples of this type of loss, which can be compounded if it is treated by oral intake of free water. Isovolemic hyponatremia is caused most commonly by the syndrome of inappropriate antidiuretic hormone (SIADH).

Table 2-2   Causes and Clinical Manifestations of Sodium Imbalance

Hyponatremia	Causes	Clinical Manifestations
	Excessive vomiting Excessive sweating Excessive water intake Adrenal insufficiency Adrenal crisis (e.g., precipitous withdrawal of corticosteroids (e.g,, prednisone [Deltasone, Orasone]) Long-term use of thiazide diuretics (e.g., metolazone [Zaroxolyn]) SIADH	*Mild hyponatremia:* Headache Fatigue Anorexia Nausea *Moderate hyponatremia:* Irritability Delirium Tachycardia Vomiting *Severe hyponatremia:* Seizures Coma
Hypernatremia	**Causes**	**Clinical Manifestations**
	Dehydration Prolonged fever Severe diarrhea Overzealous use of hypertonic saline Overzealous use of osmotic diuretics (e.g., mannitol [Osmotrol]) Cushing disease Cushing syndrome Diabetes insipidus (DI)	*Mild hypernatremia:* Fatigue *Moderate hypernatremia:* Weakness Flushed skin Low-grade fever *Severe hypernatremia:* Seizures Coma

6 Hyponatremic conditions typically are treated by treating the underlying cause first. However, patients who exhibit signs or symptoms of hyponatremia typically have dangerously low serum sodium levels that are less than 120 mEq/L and may benefit from I.V. infusion of either saline or hypertonic saline.[13] These patients must be monitored carefully because rebound cerebral edema may occur. Loop diuretics such as furosemide (Lasix) are frequently administered intravenously concomitant with the hypertonic saline to help prevent cerebral edema.[8] Treatment is halted when the serum sodium level reaches 125–130 mEq/L.[13]

HYPERNATREMIA

5 *Hypernatremia* is defined as occurring when serum sodium levels exceed 145 mEq/L. Common causes and clinical manifestations of hypernatremia are listed in Table 2-2. The most common cause of hypernatremia is dehydration, which may result from persistent diarrhea or vomiting, severe burn injuries, and excessive use of diuretics, particularly osmotic diuretics.[13] **6** Treatment tends to revolve around treating the underlying cause. I.V. treatment is not commonly indicated because oral rehydration is the preferred first-line treatment in most cases.[8] In instances where patients cannot tolerate oral rehydration, I.V. hypotonic saline solutions may be indicated for treatment. These patients also may suffer from cerebral edema if they are rehydrated too quickly, and therefore, the infusion must proceed slowly and be accompanied by careful monitoring. In general, it is recommended that half the calculated required volume of hypotonic saline should be administered over the first 24 hours, with the balance infused over the following 72 hours. The infusion generally is stopped when serum laboratory results indicate that the patient's sodium level has reached the lower limit of normal, or 145 mEq/L.[13]

Chloride Balance

4 Chloride concentration in serum mirrors that of sodium in that sodium and chloride tend to bind as salt in solution. Therefore, it is most typical that when hyponatremia occurs, so does hypochloremia, and in cases of hypernatremia, hyperchloremia also exists. **6** Therefore, treatment for hypochloremia and hyperchloremia mirrors the treatment for either hyponatremia or hypernatremia, respectively. Normal serum chloride levels range from 95 to 106 mEq/L. As noted previously, chloride is the primary extracellular anion, and its role in maintaining homeostasis largely supplements the role of sodium, but it also plays its own key role in maintaining acid–base balance.

HYPOCHLOREMIA

5 *Hypochloremia* is defined as a serum chloride level of less than 95 mEq/L. Common causes and clinical manifestations of hypochloremia are listed in Table 2-3. Hypochloremia is accompanied most frequently by hyponatremia and therefore shares the same causative factors and clinical manifestations as hyponatremia. However, chloride can bond readily not only with sodium but also with hydrogen ion (H^+). When this occurs, hydrochloric acid (HCl) forms. Thus, when metabolic alkalosis occurs because of a loss of hydrogen ion, there also may be a concomitant loss of chloride. The patient with metabolic alkalosis and hypochloremia therefore may breathe slowly and shallowly in an effort to compensate and correct the alkalosis by retaining carbon dioxide, which in water or serum can form carbonic acid, resulting in respiratory acidosis.

HYPERCHLOREMIA

5 *Hyperchloremia* occurs when the serum chloride level exceeds 106 mEq/L. Common causes and clinical manifestations of hyperchloremia are listed in Table 2-3. Hyperchloremia is a frequent consequence of hypernatremia and also shares the same causative factors and clinical manifestations. However, in instances where metabolic acidosis occurs and there is an excess of hydrogen ion, there also may be a concomitant increase in chloride levels because the two ions frequently

Table 2-3   Causes and Clinical Manifestations of Chloride Imbalance

Hypochloremia	Causes	Clinical Manifestations
	Hyponatremia Metabolic alkalosis	Same as signs and symptoms of hyponatremia (see Table 2-2) *Severe hypochloremia:* Tetany Bradypnea Respiratory acidosis Respiratory failure
Hyperchloremia	**Causes**	**Clinical Manifestations**
	Hypernatremia Metabolic acidosis	Same as signs and symptoms of hypernatremia (see Table 2-2) *Severe hyperchloremia:* Tachypnea Respiratory alkalosis Respiratory failure

bind to form HCl. The patient with metabolic acidosis and hyperchloremia therefore may exhibit tachypnea that reflects an effort to compensate by blowing off carbon dioxide, resulting in respiratory alkalosis.

Potassium Balance

4 Potassium is the major intracellular cation. Indeed, intracellular potassium levels exceed extracellular levels by over 30 times. Normal serum potassium levels are approximately 3.5–5.0 mEq/L. Potassium has an important role in ensuring appropriate cardiac cellular excitability as well as skeletal and smooth muscle contraction.[14] Because cardiac, skeletal, and smooth muscle cells are exquisitely sensitive to the influences of potassium, seemingly minor deviations from normal serum levels may have major impacts on normal cellular behavior, particularly cardiac cellular excitability and impulse conduction.

HYPOKALEMIA

5 *Hypokalemia* occurs when serum potassium levels are less than 3.5 mEq/L and is evidenced by depressed cardiac excitability and decreased smooth and skeletal muscle contraction. Because the body cannot store potassium, gastrointestinal loss of potassium through vomiting or diarrhea can rapidly cause hypokalemia. In addition, because the renal tubules excrete excess dietary potassium, use of loop diuretics also may accentuate potassium tubular excretion and cause hypokalemia. These and other etiologies and clinical manifestations of hypokalemia are listed in Table 2-4. The earliest clinical manifestation of hypokalemia is an asymptomatic depression of the T wave on the electrocardiogram (ECG). A typical ECG complex for a patient with hypokalemia is compared with a normal ECG complex in Fig. 2-3.

6 First-line treatment of hypokalemia revolves around administration of oral potassium supplements as the most effective and least costly treatment. However, many patients cannot tolerate oral potassium agents. These patients may need to receive potassium supplemental agents intravenously. Because of its profound effects on cardiac excitability, I.V. potassium must be administered cautiously, and patients treated thus should be placed on continuous cardiac monitoring. Potassium never may be administered by I.V. push or by bolus doses. Rather, potassium should be admixed with an I.V. solution and administered by an infusion controller or electronic infusion device (i.e., I.V. pump) at a rate not to exceed 10 mEq/h. In cases where a patient is severely hypokalemic and the infusion can be administered via a central line, then the administration rate may be increased to 20 mEq/h.

Table 2-4 Causes and Clinical Manifestations of Potassium Imbalance

Hypokalemia	Causes	Clinical Manifestations
	Vomiting Diarrhea Use of loop diuretics (e.g., furosemide [Lasix]) Cushing disease Cushing syndrome Heart failure Hypercalcemia Hypomagnesemia Metabolic alkalosis Aldosteronism	*Mild hypokalemia:* Flat T wave on ECG *Moderate hypokalemia:* Fatigue Lethargy Muscle cramps Orthostasis Hypotension Tachycardia U-wave development on ECG Paresthesias Hyporeflexia *Severe hypokalemia:* Paralytic ileus Coma Ventricular fibrillation Cardiopulmonary arrest
Hyperkalemia	**Causes**	**Clinical Manifestations**
	Renal failure Overzealous use of potassium supplements Rhabdomyolysis Severe burns Malignant hyperthermia Metabolic acidosis Adrenal insufficiency Adrenal crisis (e.g., precipitous withdrawal of corticosteroids [e.g., prednisone [Deltasone, Orasone]]) Tumor lysis syndrome	*Mild hyperkalemia:* Peaked T wave on ECG Paresthesias *Moderate hyperkalemia:* Irritability Nausea Diarrhea Tachycardia Palpitations *Severe hyperkalemia:* Muscle flaccidity Heart block Ventricular fibrillation Cardiopulmonary arrest

It is preferred that the primary I.V. solution does not contain dextrose because infusion of dextrose may cause the pancreas to produce more insulin. Insulin has proactive effects on the sodium–potassium pump, and more serum potassium may enter the ICF, thereby exacerbating the hypokalemia.[14]

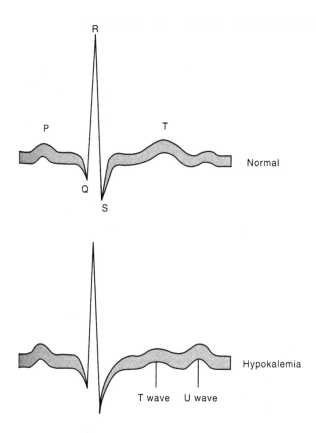

Figure 2-3   A normal ECG as compared with an ECG from a patient with hypokalemia. (Reprinted with permission from Nowak TJ, Handford AG: *Essentials of Pathophysiology: Concepts and Applications for Health Care Professionals*, 2nd ed. Boston: WCB/ McGraw-Hill, 1999:417.)

HYPERKALEMIA

5 Patients with serum potassium levels that exceed 5.0 mEq/L are *hyperkalemic*. Since the renal tubules play a key role in excreting excessive dietary potassium, their failure frequently results in hyperkalemia. Ingestion of too much potassium, particularly oral potassium supplements, is another frequent culprit that causes hyperkalemia. Any conditions that cause widespread cellular destruction, including severe burns, rhabdomyolysis, and malignant hyperthermia, result in spillage of cellular contents, including potassium, into the ECF space, causing hyperkalemia.[15] These and other causes and common clinical manifestations of hyperkalemia are listed in Table 2-4. One of the earliest classic signs of hyperkalemia includes peaking of the T wave on the ECG (Fig. 2-4).

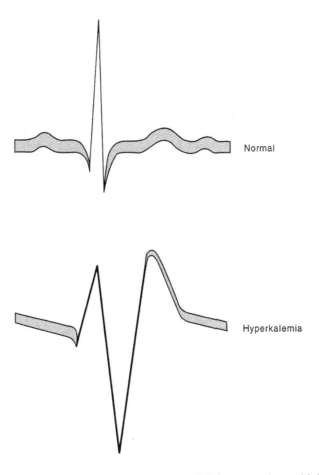

Normal

Hyperkalemia

Figure 2-4 A normal ECG as compared with an ECG from a patient with hyperkalemia. (Reprinted with permission from Nowak TJ, Handford AG: *Essentials of Pathophysiology: Concepts and Applications for Health Care Professionals*, 2nd ed. Boston: WCB/ McGraw-Hill, 1999:417.)

Sometimes the laboratory may inaccurately report a high potassium level on the serum chemistry results. This may happen if the laboratory specimen is obtained or transported traumatically, causing destruction of red blood cells (i.e., hemolysis), and will result in a falsely high serum potassium level. This is referred to as *pseudohyperkalemia*. This may be suspected when a specimen result seems high for no clearly identifiable reason, and the patient appears asymptomatic. In these instances, it is advisable to either call the laboratory to determine if the original specimen was hemolyzed or submit a second specimen for confirmatory analysis.[15]

6 Patients who are hyperkalemic with levels higher than 5.6 mEq/L or who exhibit any clinical manifestations of hyperkalemia are candidates for I.V. therapy. These patients must be placed on continuous cardiac monitors. One of the mainstays of the treatment of hyperkalemia is administering dextrose and insulin as an I.V. push. As noted previously, insulin facilitates the sodium–potassium pump, thereby drawing more potassium into the ICF compartment and out of the ECF compartment. However, insulin must be administered in conjunction with dextrose, or hypoglycemia may ensue. I.V. calcium gluconate (10%) is an agent that might be tried to stabilize the electrical activity of the heart. Finally, an infusion of sodium bicarbonate at a rate not to exceed 50 mEq/h can have the effect of pulling hydrogen ion (H+) out of the ICF and into the ECF, causing additional potassium to be pulled into the ICF compartment.[15]

SPEED BUMP

The earliest clinical manifestation of hyperkalemia is a _____ on the ECG.

Magnesium Balance

4 Magnesium levels normally range between 1.3 and to 2.2 mEq/L. Magnesium is important in ensuring activation of enzymes, in regulating DNA and RNA synthesis, in stabilizing the sodium–potassium pump, and in maintaining calcium channel activity.

HYPOMAGNESEMIA

5 *Hypomagnesemia* occurs when the serum concentration of magnesium is less than 1.3 mEq/L. It occurs most commonly when there is poor magnesium dietary intake or absorption or when there is accelerated magnesium excretion in the urine, as may happen when many different types of diuretics are administered.[8] Because hypocalcemia is a frequent concomitant occurrence, the clinical manifestations of hypomagnesemia are similar to those of hypocalcemia (compare Tables 2-5 and 2-6). **6** Treatment revolves around providing magnesium supplements, either orally or parenterally.

HYPERMAGNESEMIA

5 *Hypermagnesemia* is defined as a serum concentration of magnesium of more than 2.2 mEq/L. It ensues most commonly as a result of renal failure or because of ingestion of too much magnesium-based antacid. Because magnesium inhibits the release of acetylcholine at neural junctions, progressive clinical manifestations are consistent with widespread smooth and skeletal muscle flaccidity and their eventual nonresponsiveness. This results in eventual cardiac and respiratory failure. Common causes and clinical manifestations of hypermagnesemia are displayed on Table 2-5.

Table 2-5   Causes and Clinical Manifestations of Magnesium Imbalance

Hypomagnesemia	Causes	Clinical Manifestations
	Malnutrition Alcoholism Severe diarrhea Overzealous use of diuretics	*Mild hypomagnesemia:* Hyperreflexia Weakness *Moderate hypomagnesemia:* Vertigo Ataxia Nystagmus Paresthesias Tremors Tetany Seizures Hypertension Paralytic ileus Abdominal cramps *Severe hypermagnesemia:* Dysrhythmias Status epilepticus Cardiopulmonary arrest
Hypermagnesemia	**Causes**	**Clinical Manifestations**
	Renal failure Overzealous use of magnesium-based antacids (e.g., magnesium hydroxide [milk of magnesia]) Adrenal insufficiency Adrenal crisis Lithium toxicity	*Mild hypermagnesemia:* Hyporeflexia Lethargy *Moderate hypermagnesemia:* Areflexia Flushing Diaphoresis Vomiting Muscle flaccidity *Severe hypermagnesemia:* Diplopia Heart block Hypotension Bradypnea Cardiopulmonary arrest

6 I.V. hydration to accelerate magnesium renal excretion may be indicated to treat hypermagnesemia. I.V. push calcium gluconate may be administered because calcium antagonizes the effects of magnesium. In patients with either severe hypermagnesemia or renal failure, hemodialysis may be indicated to filter and excrete excess magnesium.[13]

Calcium Balance

4 Normal serum calcium levels range between 4.5 and 5.5 mEq/L. Calcium is the primary electrolyte that provides the matrix for bones. It also plays a vital role in ensuring appropriate muscular contraction and transmission of neural impulses. In addition, it behaves as a clotting factor in the clotting cascade and therefore has a key role in ensuring that hemostatic function is maintained.

HYPOCALCEMIA

5 *Hypocalcemia* is defined as a serum calcium level of less than 4.5 mEq/L. Hypocalcemia may be caused by an inadequate intake of calcium-rich foods or by an inadequacy in vitamin D levels, which is necessary to ensure proper absorption of calcium. A loss in parathyroid hormone, which acts by mobilizing calcium stores, may cause hypocalcemia, as can accelerated renal excretion of calcium, which may occur when loop diuretics are used. Injuries and diseases that cause widespread necrosis can cause hypocalcemia because calcium tends to bind to necrotic tissue. Common causes and clinical manifestations of hypocalcemia are listed in Table 2-6. **6** Treatment tends to revolve around administration of calcium supplements, with the oral route preferred. If the patient is severely hypocalcemic or symptomatic, an I.V. infusion of calcium may be indicated in the form of calcium gluconate or calcium chloride.[8]

HYPERCALCEMIA

5 Hypercalcemia occurs when the serum calcium level exceeds 5.5 mEq/L. Many patients who are hypercalcemic are frail and chronically ill. They may be on prolonged bed rest, causing depletion of calcium from the bony matrix, or they may have malignant neoplasms that cause hypercalcemia. Other causes of hypercalcemia include an excessive intake of either calcium or vitamin D and hyperparathyroidism.[8]

Additional causes and clinical manifestations of hypercalcemia are displayed on Table 2-6. **6** The most common treatment indicated for hypercalcemia is hydration therapy. I.V. hydration may be indicated in patients who cannot tolerate oral fluids and may be accompanied by calcitonin and I.V. push loop diuretics such as furosemide (Lasix) to accelerate renal excretion of calcium.[13]

Table 2-6 Causes and Clinical Manifestations of Calcium Imbalance

Hypocalcemia	Causes	Clinical Manifestations
	Inadequate oral intake of calcium or vitamin D Hypoparathyroidism Hyperphosphatemia Overzealous use of loop diuretics (e.g., Furosemide [Lasix]) Pancreatitis Severe burns Alkalosis	*Mild hypocalcemia:* Fatigue Muscle cramps in extremities *Moderate hypocalcemia:* Paresthesias, particularly perioral Abdominal cramps Widespread muscle cramps Hyperreflexia Carpal spasm (i.e., Trousseau sign) Facial spasm (i.e., Chvostek sign) *Severe hypocalcemia:* Tetany Seizures Laryngospasm Prolonged QT interval on ECG Dysrhythmias Cardiopulmonary arrest
Hypercalcemia	**Causes**	**Clinical Manifestations**
	Excessive oral intake of calcium or vitamin D Hyperparathyroidism Prolonged bed rest Hypophosphatemia Overzealous use of thiazide diuretics (e.g., chlorothiazide [Diuril]) Lithium toxicity Malignant neoplasms Adrenal insufficiency Adrenal crisis	*Mild hypercalcemia:* Nausea Thirst Anorexia Fatigue *Moderate hypercalcemia:* Confusion Hyporeflexia Polyuria Polydipsia Weakness Muscle flaccidity *Severe hypercalcemia:* Coma Heart block Shortened QT interval on ECG Dysrhythmias Cardiopulmonary arrest

Phosphate Balance

4 Typical serum phosphorus levels range from 2.5–4.5 mEq/L. Phosphorus has an important role in maintaining ATP stores, shares a role with calcium in maintaining bone matrix, and aids in the metabolism of nutrients. Phosphorus levels tend to behave in a manner that is reciprocal to calcium levels. That is, hypocalcemia is commonly concomitant with hyperphosphatemia, and when hypercalcemia occurs, hypophosphatemia typically occurs in tandem. Table 2-7 displays common causes and clinical manifestations of both hypophosphatemia and hyperphosphatemia.

HYPOPHOSPHATEMIA

5 *Hypophosphatemia* occurs when the serum phosphorus level drops below 2.5 mEq/L. It occurs most frequently when hypercalcemia occurs. It also may occur in patients who are treated successfully for diabetic ketoacidosis (DKA) with insulin because phosphorus may be pulled into the cells as a result of insulin's effect on the cellular membrane. **6** I.V. phosphorus supplements may be prescribed for patients who are severely hypophosphatemic or who exhibit clinical manifestations of hypophosphatemia. In these instances, the supplemental infusion should proceed slowly with frequent monitoring of both the serum phosphorus levels and the serum calcium levels because hypocalcemia may result if too much phosphorus is administered.[8]

Table 2-7 Causes and Clinical Manifestations of Phosphate Imbalance

Hypophosphatemia	Causes	Clinical Manifestations
	Hypercalcemia Resolving DKA Overzealous use of antacids	Same as signs and symptoms of hypercalcemia (see Table 2-6)
Hyperphosphatemia	**Causes**	**Clinical Manifestations**
	Hypocalcemia Renal failure Rhabdomyolysis Tumor lysis syndrome	Same as signs and symptoms of hypocalcemia (see Table 2-6)

HYPERPHOSPHATEMIA

5 Phosphorus levels in excess of 4.5 mEq/L are consistent with *hyperphospha-temia.* Hypocalcemia is a frequent concomitant occurrence. It also is a frequent consequence of renal failure. **6** The treatment for hyperphosphatemia is the same as for hypocalcemia because low serum calcium levels carry more serious conse-quences than does an excess of phosphorus.

Summary

Fluid and electrolytes perform vital functions in maintaining homeostasis. Understanding the composition of fluid and electrolytes in body fluid compartments, their homeostatic mechanisms, and the role of key electrolytes in maintaining the function of these fluid compartments and in maintaining metabolic function is requisite to understanding indications for I.V. therapy.

Quiz

1. Which of the following patients is *least* susceptible to dehydration?

    (a) An obese middle-age female

    (b) A normal-sized, healthy adult male

    (c) An elderly but healthy male

    (d) A normal-sized, healthy 12-month-old infant

2. The majority of body fluids can be found in which compartment?

    (a) Intracellular

    (b) Extracellular

    (c) Interstitium

    (d) Intravascular

3. Which of the following is the major determinant of colloidal osmotic pressure (COP) within the intravascular compartment?

(a) Sodium

(b) Potassium

(c) Fibrinogen

(d) Albumin

4. Movement of water across a semipermeable membrane from an area with a lesser concentration of solute to an area with a greater concentration of solute is the definition of

(a) diffusion.

(b) osmosis.

(c) the port system.

(d) the pump system.

5. Aldosterone facilitates renal reabsorption of which of the following electrolytes?

(a) Sodium

(b) Chloride

(c) Potassium

(d) Magnesium

6. A cell would shrink if it were placed in a bath of which of the following types of solutions?

(a) Isotonic

(b) Hypotonic

(c) Hypertonic

(d) Saline

7. Which type of condition can cause hyperchloremia?

(a) Metabolic alkalosis

(b) Metabolic acidosis

(c) Respiratory alkalosis

(d) Respiratory acidosis

8. What is the recommended intravenous infusion rate of potassium in a patient who is hypokalemic?

    (a) No more than 10 mEq/h in an admixed solution. If a central I.V. line is used, no more than 20 mEq/h

    (b) No more than 20 mEq by I.V. push

    (c) No more than 50 mEq in a bolus dose

    (d) No more than 10 mEq in a central I.V. line bolus

9. Treatment of hyperphosphatemia typically involves

    (a) rehydration I.V. therapy.

    (b) potassium I.V. boluses.

    (c) hemodialysis.

    (d) hypocalcemia treatment.

CHAPTER 3

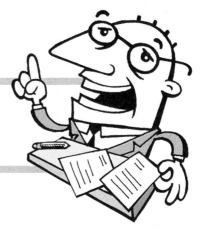

Intravenous Therapy Delivery Systems

Learning Objectives

After completing this chapter, the learner will

1. Describe features of commonly used intravenous (I.V.) therapy containers, including glass bottles and plastic bags.

2. Define common terms used in describing the setup of I.V. administration sets, including spiking and priming.

3. Compare and contrast indications for use of primary and secondary infusion sets.

4. Identify indications for use of mechanical and electronic infusion delivery systems.

5 Accurately calculate I.V. drip rates when given a specific I.V. administration prescription and a specific type of I.V. administration set.

6 Describe features commonly available in many electronic infusion devices.

 Key Terms

Luer locks

Spiking

Primary infusion sets

Secondary infusion sets

Extension sets

Priming

Drop factor

Macrodrop sets

Microdrop sets

Introduction to Intravenous (I.V.) Therapy Delivery Systems

The nurse must be comfortable working with commonly used I.V. therapy equipment in order to ensure that the patient receives the infusion of fluids, blood components, medications, or nutrients that is prescribed by the physician or the advanced-practice clinician with prescriptive authority authorized by his or her respective governing state board of nursing or medicine. An advanced-practice clinician who has this type of authorization may include a nurse practitioner, nurse midwife, nurse anesthetist, or physician assistant.

Any infusion delivered to a patient by the I.V. route must be sterile, or pathogens that are introduced may cause septicemia. Therefore, all connecting ports between I.V. containers, lines, filters, and access devices must remain secure and sterile. It is not necessary that the nurse wear gloves when setting up an administration set. However, the nurse must wash his or her hands thoroughly and vigorously prior to setting up an I.V. administration set and must be careful not to touch or otherwise contaminate open ports or tips before they are connected into the system. Connectors known as **Luer locks** are advocated because they provide a secure screw-type connection between connecting I.V. lines and hubs of I.V. access devices.[6] Taping interconnecting parts of the I.V. administration setup, though performed commonly in years past, is not advocated.[6]

Infusion Containers

1 Intravenous infusion containers come in a variety of sizes that range from 50 to over 2000 mL. One liter (i.e., 1000 mL) is the most common I.V. infusion container size employed for infusion of the most frequently used I.V. solutions, which are called *crystalloids* and are discussed in Chapter 7. **2** The nurse should visually inspect the I.V. infusion container prior to **spiking** it with an infusion set. Spiking an I.V. container with an infusion set means that the sterile tip of the infusion set has penetrated the seal of the container. If the solution appears discolored, not of uniform color, or contains any particulate matter, the container is discarded. The container should not be cracked or otherwise appear violated, or it likewise should be discarded.

SPEED BUMP

_____ an I.V. container with an infusion set means that the sterile tip of the infusion set has penetrated the seal of the container.

There are two types of I.V. infusion containers—glass bottles and plastic bags. No matter which type of container is used, and no matter whether or not an infusion pump is used to aid in the precise delivery of the prescribed solution, it is good practice to adhere a time tape to the side of the container. The time tape at a minimum should note the time and date that the container was spiked (or accessed by an I.V. infusion set), the initials of the nurse who spiked the container, and incremental markings that denote approximate times that solution should empty from the container. If there is a change in order of the delivery rate of the solution, then the time tape also should be altered to reflect this change.

GLASS I.V. BOTTLES

Glass I.V. bottles were the first closed types of I.V. containers used. They tend to not be used as frequently as plastic I.V. bags for delivery of most solutions today because they are harder to store and easier to crack. Glass I.V. bottles are indicated for admixing medications and nutrients that might interact with the plastics commonly used in plastic I.V. bags. Examples of admixtures that are known to interact with plastic include nitroglycerin and fat emulsions.[16]

Glass I.V. bottles feature a rubber disk plug that is covered by a sterile seal. After the seal is removed, the rubber disk is penetrated with the sterile tip, or spike, of the I.V. infusion set. The bottles are vacuum-packed, so air must be permitted to flow into the bottle to displace the solution. If the bottle is packed so that it contains a venting straw, then airflow is already ensured. If the bottle does not contain a venting straw, then a vented I.V. infusion set must be selected or flow of solution

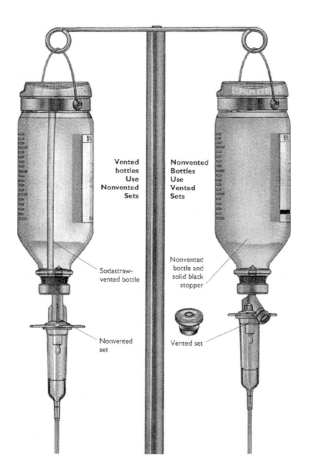

Figure 3-1   Vented and nonvented glass I.V. bottles. (Used with permission from Perucca R: Infusion therapy equipment: Types of infusion therapy equipment. In Hankins J, Lonsway RAW, Hedrick C, Perdue MB (eds.): *The Infusion Nurses Society: Infusion Therapy in Clinical Practice,* 2nd ed. Philadelphia: Saunders, 2001, Fig. 15-1.)

from the bottle will not occur.[16] Figure 3-1 displays vented and nonvented glass bottles with respective nonvented and vented tubing. The glass bottle is spiked with an appropriate I.V. infusion set after the tubing is clamped, and the bottle then is hung on an I.V. pole as displayed in the figure.

PLASTIC I.V. BAGS

Plastic I.V. bags are the most commonly used I.V. containers because they are easy to store and less vulnerable to damage than glass containers. Figure 3-2 shows a variety of plastic I.V. bags. Because these plastic bags can collapse, they do not need to be vented to ensure flow of solution from the bag into the I.V. infusion set. These bags contain an

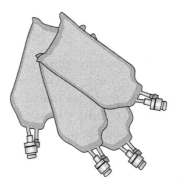

Figure 3-2   Intravenous bags.

access port with a sterile sheath. When the sterile sheath is removed, the access port of the bag is spiked with the tip of the I.V. infusion set after the clamp on the infusion set is closed, as displayed in Figure 3-3. The I.V. bag then is hung on an I.V. pole.

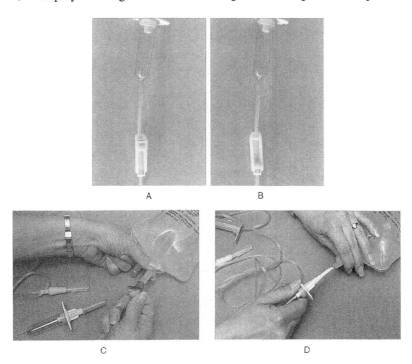

Figure 3-3   Steps in spiking an I.V. bag with a primary infusion set. *A.* Roller camp is packed open. *B.* Roller clamp is closed. *C.* Protective sheath is removed from I.V. bag port. *D.* Protective cap is removed from the spike, and the spike is inserted into the I.V. bag. (Used with permission from Perry AG, Potter PA: *Clinical Nursing Skills and Techniques,* 5th ed. St. Louis: Mosby, 2002:568.)

I.V. Lines

3 Intravenous lines can include primary infusion sets, secondary infusion sets, and extension sets. Primary and secondary infusion sets both contain spikes and drip chambers, whereas extension sets do not contain spikes or drip chambers. The I.V. tubing on both infusion sets and extension sets can be of a variety of lengths and may contain one or several clamps and one or several injection or access ports.

PRIMARY INFUSION SETS

A **primary infusion set** is the main tubing that carries continuously infusing solution from the I.V. bag or bottle into the patient's vein by way of a venous access device. Peripheral venous access devices are described in Chapter 4, and central venous access devices are described in Chapter 5. Primary infusion sets vary in length from 60 to 110 inches. Minimum characteristics of these sets include a spike to access the I.V. bag or bottle, a drip chamber, and at least one clamp. The clamp is typically a roller clamp, although a slide clamp or a screw clamp could be used.

Most primary infusion sets also feature one or more injection ports or injection sites that may be used to inject medications by either "piggyback" infusion or I.V. push. Injection ports typically are designed so that they may be accessed by either needleless injection devices or by needle-protected devices so that the risk of needlestick injury is minimized. The end of the tubing that is distal to the spike typically features a Luer lock design so that the likelihood of disconnection from the hub of the I.V. access device is minimized.[16] Figure 3-4 shows two types of primary I.V. administration sets.

SECONDARY INFUSION SETS

Secondary infusion sets share many of the same characteristics as primary infusion sets, including a spike, a drip chamber, one or several clamps, and sometimes one or several access ports. However, they are used for either continuous or intermittent infusion of medications that are "piggybacked" into the primary line by either a needleless injection device or a needle-protected device. The continuously infused solution delivered by the primary infusion set must be compatible with the medication delivered by the secondary infusion set. Secondary infusion sets tend to be shorter than primary infusion sets and are commonly designed at 30–36 inches in length.[16]

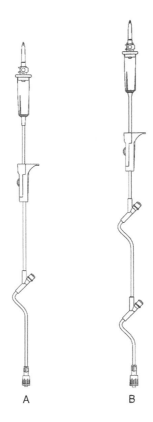

A   B

Figure 3-4 Primary I.V. administration setups. *A.* Primary I.V. administration setup with one injection port. *B.* Primary I.V. administration setup with two injection ports. (Courtesy of B. Braun, Products Catalog, 2005).

EXTENSION SETS

Extension sets may be used when additional length or injection ports are needed on an I.V. administration setup. These sets are rarely indicated today as compared with years past because there are many more manufacturers' choices for selecting primary infusion sets of a number of lengths that contain additional access ports and clamps. Adding an extension set to an I.V. delivery system carries an additional risk of system disconnection and contamination, even when Luer-lock devices are used. Therefore, their general use is discouraged.[16] Figure 3-5 shows common extension sets.

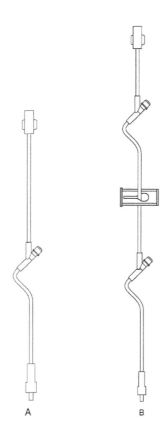

Figure 3-5 Extension I.V. sets. *A.* Extension set with one injection port. *B.* Extension set with two injection ports and one slide clamp. (Courtesy of B. Braun, Products Catalog, 2005.)

PRIMING I.V. LINES

2 Priming an I.V. line means that the prescribed solution is uniformly flushed through the I.V. administration setup. After the I.V. bag or bottle is spiked with the administration set and placed on the I.V. pole, as described previously, the solution must be uniformly flushed through the line before the line is attached to the venous access device and before the solution is infused into the patient. To accomplish this, the drip chamber of the administration set is squeezed as demonstrated in Fig. 3-6 until it is approximately one-third to one-half filled with I.V. solution. If too little solution is squeezed into the chamber, the chamber may be squeezed repeatedly until the desired amount of fluid is present in the chamber. If too much solution fills the chamber, the bag or bottle may be inverted, and some solution may be squeezed back into the bag or bottle.

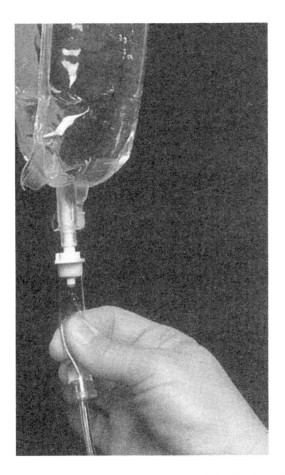

Figure 3-6   Demonstration of technique to squeeze the drip chamber. (Used with permission from Perry AG, Potter PA: *Clinical Nursing Skills and Techniques,* 5th ed. St. Louis: Mosby, 2002:569.)

SPEED BUMP

_____ *an I.V. line means that the prescribed solution is uniformly flushed through the I.V. administration setup.*

Once the drip chamber is filled to an appropriate level with solution, the cap on the distal end of the tubing is removed and set aside. The end of the cap that interfaces with the tubing is kept sterile. The I.V. tubing then is held taut, and the clamp is partially unclamped so that solution flows slowly through the I.V. line. Holding the line taut and only permitting the solution to flow slowly minimize the formation of air bubbles. The line is inspected for the formation of air bubbles, which may be flushed slowly out of the line with the administration solution.

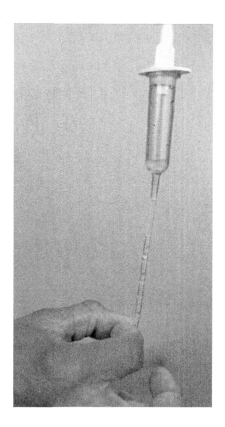

Figure 3-7   Demonstration of removal of air bubbles from I.V. tubing. (Used with permission from Perry AG, Potter PA: *Clinical Nursing Skills and Techniques,* 5th ed. St. Louis: Mosby, 2002:568.)

Alternatively, the line may be held taut and gently tapped with a finger, encouraging air bubbles to flow upward and eventually back into the drip chamber. Figure 3-7 demonstrates this technique. Once the I.V. line is primed with solution and the line is thoroughly inspected and found to be free from air bubbles, then the I.V. line cap is placed back on the end of the I.V. tubing using sterile technique. The cap remains in place until the I.V. administration setup is connected to the I.V. access device.

Delivering I.V. Solutions

Solutions that infuse through I.V. administration sets may be titrated at approximate drip rates by setting appropriate tension or pressure on the administration set's roller clamp, or they may be programmed to infuse at a set rate by a flow-rate control device or an electronic infusion device. The most accurate way to deliver an infusion rate via an I.V. administration set is by using an electronic infusion device.

4 In general, when it is necessary to deliver a consistent rate of a given solution accurately, an electronic infusion device, such as an I.V. pump, is indicated. Most continuously infused medications and many intermittently infused, "piggybacked" medications must be infused via secondary infusion sets by means of an I.V. pump. Although it is not absolutely necessary to deliver all intermittently infused, "piggybacked" medications or all solutions by the primary infusion set through an I.V. pump, it is preferred to use this type of setup if the equipment is available because there are fewer complications associated with using an I.V. pump. It is much easier to ensure that a patient receives an accurately dosed volume of solution over a given period of time using an I.V. pump. Alternatively, if an I.V. pump is not available, flow-rate control devices that are, in essence, mechanical dials placed on the I.V. administration set can be used to deliver reasonably accurate volumes of solution.

Infusing primary solutions such as crystalloids without an I.V. pump or other control device requires that the solution drains by gravity, and the administration rate is titrated by placing varying amounts of tension or pressure on the I.V. line via the roller clamp or the screw clamp on the administration set. A slide clamp cannot be used for this purpose. The rate of infusion of the I.V. solution may vary over time by a considerable amount based on position of the I.V. tubing and position of the patient's arm. It is very easy to inadvertently deliver unnecessary boluses of I.V. fluids or less than adequate amounts of solution because of a simple change of position of the administration setup. Intravenous pump rates do not change based on changes in position of the administration setup, and therefore, I.V. pumps are much more likely to deliver consistent amounts of solution to the patient. Nonetheless, it is still important for the nurse to be capable of calculating I.V. drip rates by gravity infusion of administration setups in the event that I.V. pumps are not available for use.

CALCULATING I.V. DRIP RATES

5 Continuously infused I.V. solution drip rates are calculated based on the amount of solution to be infused each hour. The formula for this type of calculation is

Total infusion volume ordered/total infusion time in hours = rate of solution/hour

For instance, if an order for an I.V. solution specifies that a patient is to receive 2 L (2000 mL) of solution in 16 hours, then the patient's hourly rate of infusion is calculated as follows:

2000 mL (total infusion volume)/16 h (total infusion time) = 125 mL/h

And if an order for an I.V. solution specifies that a patient is to receive 4 L (4000 mL) of solution in 24 hours, then the patient's hourly rate of infusion is calculated as follows:

4000 mL (total infusion volume)/24 h (total infusion time) = 167 mL/h

If a patient is prescribed a bolus dose of an I.V. solution to infuse over a shortened time frame, that is, over minutes rather than hours, the minutes must be converted to fractions of hours as follows:

Total infusion time in minutes/60 min/h = infusion time in hours

For instance, if an order for an I.V. solution specifies that a patient is to receive 200 mL of solution in 10 minutes, then the first step in calculating the infusion rate necessitates converting the minutes to hours as follows:

10 min/60 min/h = 0.1667 h

Then the second step of this calculation uses the first formula, which is

Total infusion volume ordered/total infusion time in hours = rate of solution/hour

or

200 mL (total infusion volume)/0.1667 h (total infusion time) = 1200 mL/h

If an administration setup is used that is set to gravity drainage and is not set to an I.V. pump, then the drops per minute must be calculated based on the **drop factor,** or the number of drops contained in 1 mL of solution, which is noted by the manufacturer of the administration set. Drops per minute are counted as they infuse into the drip chamber over 1 minute's time. To speed up the rate of infusion, and thus the number of drops per minute, less tension or pressure is placed on the administration set clamp. To slow the rate of infusion, and thus the number of drops per minute, more tension or pressure is placed on the administration clamp.

Infusion sets are referred to as **macrodrop sets** if the drop factor is 10, 12, 15, or 20 drops/mL, and they are referred to as **microdrop sets,** or sometimes *pediatric drip sets,* if the drop factor is 50 or 60 drops/mL. Microdrop sets typically are identifiable because there is a visible needle in the middle of the drip chamber.

The formula to calculate the number of drops per minute to regulate the hourly rate of infusion of solution is

(Total infusion volume × drop factor)/total infusion time converted to minutes = drops/minute

For instance, if a patient is supposed to receive 125 mL/h of a given solution, and the administration set is a macrodrop set with a drop factor of 15 drops/mL, then the number of drops per minute that must be titrated on the administration set by applying appropriate tension on the roller clamp that is calculated as follows:

$$(125 \text{ mL/h} \times 15 \text{ drops/mL})/60 \text{ min/h} = 31.25 \text{ drops/min}$$

Because it is not possible to titrate fractions or portions of drops, convention dictates that the drops per minute are either rounded up if the calculated remainder is at least 0.50 drops and rounded down if the calculated remainder is less than 0.50 drops. Therefore, in the preceding example, the actual number of drops titrated is not 31.25 drops but 31 drops. Subsequent examples in this section will use this convention of rounding the remainder.

If a patient is prescribed to receive 200 mL/h of a given solution, and the administration set is a macrodrop set with a drop factor of 20 drops/mL, then the number of drops per minute that must be titrated, as described previously, is calculated as follows:

$$(200 \text{ mL/h} \times 20 \text{ drops/mL})/60 \text{ min/h} = 67 \text{ drops/min}$$

If a patient is supposed to receive 100 mL/h of a given solution, and the administration set is a macrodrop set with a drop factor of 12 drops/mL, then the number of drops per minute that is titrated is calculated as follows:

$$(100 \text{ mL/h} \times 12 \text{ drops/mL})/60 \text{ min/h} = 20 \text{ drops/min}$$

And if a patient is prescribed to receive 75 mL/h of solution, and the chosen macrodrop administration set has a drop factor of 10 drops/mL, then the number of drops per minute that must be titrated is calculated as follows:

$$(75 \text{ mL/h} \times 10 \text{ drops/mL})/60 \text{ min/h} = 13 \text{ drops/min}$$

If a pediatric patient is supposed to receive 50 mL/h of a given solution by a microdrip administration set with a drop factor of 60 drops/mL, then the number of drops per minute that must be titrated is calculated as follows:

$$(50 \text{ mL/h} \times 60 \text{ drops/mL})/60 \text{ min/h} = 50 \text{ drops/min}$$

Similarly, if a pediatric patient is prescribed to receive 75 mL/h of a given solution by a microdrop administration set with a drop factor of 50 drops/mL, then the number of drops per minute that must be titrated is calculated as follows:

$$(75 \text{ mL/h} \times 50 \text{ drops/mL})/60 \text{ min/h} = 63 \text{ drops/min}$$

I.V. DELIVERY DEVICES

4 There are two basic types of I.V. delivery devices—mechanical and electronic. Electronic infusion devices tend to be used much more commonly in inpatient acute-care settings, whereas mechanical infusion devices tend to be used almost exclusively in home-care settings.[16]

Mechanical Infusion Devices

TIP *Mechanical infusion devices do not rely on sources of electricity to operate. They operated based on simple principles of mechanical engineering and operate by infusing a consistent volume of solution through pressure generated either by a preinflated balloon or by a type of wound spring. Three common types of mechanical infusion devices include the elastomeric balloon, the spring-coil piston syringe, and the spring-coil container. None of these types of infusion devices is designed to deliver large volumes of solution. Typically, they can only deliver less than 100 mL of any solution.[16]*

Electronic Infusion Devices

Electronic infusion devices may include controllers and positive-pressure infusion pumps. Controllers do not regulate flow rate directly; rather, gravity is used to ensure infusion. When flow is disrupted, interrupted, or inconsistent, an alarm sounds so that the nurse may reset or troubleshoot the setup.

Positive-pressure infusion pumps are also called *I.V. pumps* and are the most commonly used I.V. delivery device. Intravenous pumps have a variety of features that ensure quality control and safety for the patient. Many I.V. pumps require their own specific type of administration set that provides proper interface with the pump equipment. Intravenous pumps can be programmed to regulate the rate of delivery of the solution within a confidence interval of 95 percent. **6** In addition, most pumps keep electronic records of the volume to be infused and the volume that has been infused over a given period of time that are readily retrievable. Some pumps have a variety of other options. Some pumps can maintain a lengthy record of historical data for infusions over a time period, whereas others can identify drug and solution incompatibilities. Some pumps can regulate an additional intermittent secondary infusion, whereas others are even more sophisticated and permit the simultaneous use of several continuous pump channels. All I.V. pumps feature alarms, which include air alarms (e.g., that may denote air in the line or disconnection), occlusion alarms, low-power alarms, and an alarm that sounds when the infusion is complete.[16] Figure 11-2 displays an I.V. pump.

There are some special types of I.V. pumps that include ambulatory pumps for use by patients in outpatient settings. These pumps are discussed in further detail in Chapter 14. Another commonly used special type of I.V. pump that is used frequently in the inpatient acute-care setting is the patient-controlled analgesia pump (PCA pump).

PCA pumps may be manufactured so that they use an I.V. bag but more frequently are designed so that they use prefilled syringes of analgesic agents. PCA pumps can be programmed so that they feature many of the same options as a standard I.V. pump. They also can be programmed so that the patient receives a *basal rate* of the analgesic agent, which refers to a certain minimum hourly rate of analgesic solution that the PCA administers, and a *demand rate,* which is an "as needed" rate (e.g., PRN dose) that the patient may receive within a given time limit by pushing a button on the device. These devices have a lock-out safety feature that means that only the patient's nurse may change the rate of infusion by inserting a key and reprogramming the PCA pump.

Summary

Some I.V. delivery systems are relatively simplistic, whereas others are fairly complex. In order to ensure safe and effective delivery of prescribed I.V. solutions, the nurse must be competent working with a variety of I.V. delivery systems. Understanding the basic principles that underlie the delivery of I.V. solutions by several commonly used systems helps to ensure this competency.

Quiz

1. Which type of connections are advocated as safest for ensuring appropriate interface between the components of an I.V. delivery system?
   (a) Taped connections
   (b) Velcro connections
   (c) Luer-lock connections
   (d) Locked connections

2. Which of the following statements regarding glass I.V. bottles is true?
   (a) They are easier to store than plastic I.V. bags.
   (b) They are less susceptible to cracking than plastic I.V. bags.
   (c) They are collapsible and so do not require venting.
   (d) They tend to be compatible with medications and solutions that interact with plastics.

3. An extension set includes which of the following?

   (a) A spike

   (b) A drip chamber

   (c) At least one clamp

   (d) Intravenous tubing

4. A microdrip infusion set may feature a drop factor of

   (a) 12 drops/mL.

   (b) 15 drops/mL.

   (c) 20 drops/mL.

   (d) 50 drops/mL

5. The physician orders that a patient receive 3000 mL of I.V. solution in 24 hours. What is the appropriate delivery rate of the solution?

   (a) 100 mL/h

   (b) 125 mL/h

   (c) 150 mL/h

   (d) 200 mL/h

6. The physician orders that a patient receive 1000 mL of I.V. solution in 8 hours. What is the appropriate delivery rate of the solution?

   (a) 100 mL/h

   (b) 125 mL/h

   (c) 150 mL/h

   (d) 200 mL/h

7. The physician orders that a patient receive a 250-mL bolus of I.V. solution in 20 minutes. What is the appropriate delivery rate of the solution?

   (a) 125 mL/h

   (b) 250 mL/h

   (c) 500 mL/h

   (d) 750 mL/h

8. A patient is to receive an I.V. solution at a rate of 150 mL/h. The I.V. administration set has a drop factor if 12 drops/mL. How many drops per minute must be titrated to achieve the prescribed infusion rate?

    (a) 17 drops/min

    (b) 30 drops/min

    (c) 31 drops/min

    (d) 42 drops/min

9. A patient is to receive an I.V. solution at a rate of 125 mL/h. The I.V. administration set has a drop factor of 20 drops/mL. How many drops per minute must be titrated to achieve the prescribed infusion rate?

    (a) 17 drops/min

    (b) 30 drops/min

    (c) 31 drops/min

    (d) 42 drops/min

10. A patient is to receive an I.V. solution at a rate of 100 mL/h. The I.V. administration set has a drop factor of 10 drops/mL. How many drops per minute must be titrated to achieve the prescribed infusion rate?

    (a) 17 drops/min

    (b) 30 drops/min

    (c) 31 drops/min

    (d) 42 drops/min

11. A pediatric patient is to receive an I.V. solution at a rate of 60 mL/h. The I.V. administration set has a drop factor of 60 drops/mL. How many drops per minute must be titrated to achieve the prescribed infusion rate?

    (a) 33 drops/min

    (b) 50 drops/min

    (c) 60 drops/min

    (d) 67 drops/min

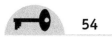

12. A pediatric patient is to receive an I.V. solution at a rate of 80 mL/h. The
    I.V. administration set has a drop factor of 50 drops/mL. How many drops
    per minute must be titrated to achieve the prescribed infusion rate?

    (a) 33 drops/min

    (b) 50 drops/min

    (c) 60 drops/min

    (d) 67 drops/min

13. A pediatric patient is to receive an I.V. solution at a rate of 40 mL/h. The
    I.V. administration set has a drop factor of 50 drops/mL. How many drops
    per minute must be titrated to achieve the prescribed infusion rate?

    (a) 33 drops/min

    (b) 50 drops/min

    (c) 60 drops/min

    (d) 67 drops/min

14. A pediatric patient is to receive an I.V. solution at a rate of 50 mL/h. The
    I.V. administration set has a drop factor of 60 drops/mL. How many drops
    per minute must be titrated to achieve the prescribed infusion rate?

    (a) 33 drops/min

    (b) 50 drops/min

    (c) 60 drops/min

    (d) 67 drops/min

15. Intravenous pumps

    (a) feature a variety of alarms.

    (b) flow by gravity.

    (c) can interface with most standard I.V. administration sets.

    (d) use a spring-coil mechanism.

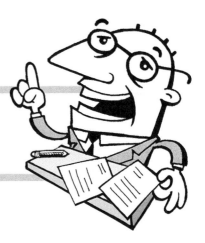

CHAPTER 4

Peripheral Intravenous Therapy

Learning Objectives

After completing this chapter, the learner will

1   Discuss common indications for initiating and maintaining peripheral intravenous (I.V.) therapy.

2   Understand the steps required to initiate a peripheral I.V. line.

3   Differentiate between commonly used peripheral venous access devices in terms of their physical features and their indications for use.

4   Identify methods that may provide stability to an I.V. access device.

5   Describe the steps required to change an I.V. infusion setup, to change an I.V. access site dressing, and to discontinue an I.V. administration setup.

Key Terms

Steel-winged infusion devices	Midline catheters
Over-the-needle catheters	Saline locks
Short catheters	

Indications for Peripheral Intravenous (I.V.) Therapy

1 The most common indication for initiating I.V. therapy by a peripheral venous access route is to treat or prevent fluid and electrolyte disturbances. In these instances, the infusion fluids of choice typically are types of solutions referred to as *crystalloids*. Less commonly selected types of infusion fluids could be *colloids*. Indications for selecting common crystalloid and colloid solutions are discussed in Chapters 7 and 8, respectively.

Initiating peripheral I.V. therapy also may be indicated to replace or supplement blood components. Indications for administering common blood components are discussed in Chapter 9. Another common indication for initiating I.V. therapy is to administer medications by the I.V. route, including intermittently administered medications (e.g., I.V. push medications, I.V. "piggyback" medications) and continuously infused medications, which are described in more detail in Chapter 11. In general, if the patient has a central I.V. access device in place, it is preferred to administer blood components and many medications by the central route rather than peripherally. Indications for central I.V. therapy are discussed in Chapter 5. However, if the patient does not have a central I.V. access device already in place, peripheral routes frequently are considered sufficient for achieving the intended therapeutic effect simply because there are more inherent risks associated with initiating and maintaining central I.V. venous access routes than peripheral I.V. access routes.

A much less common indication for initiating I.V. therapy by a peripheral route is to deliver peripheral parenteral nutrition. Central I.V. lines are indicated most commonly as the vascular delivery route for parenteral nutrients, and this is discussed in more detail in Chapter 10. It is generally not possible to infuse sufficient daily caloric requirements for most patients through the peripheral route, but this is possible to achieve via the central route.

Initiating I.V. Therapy

Prior to initiating I.V. therapy, the nurse must verify that an appropriate prescriptive order has been written by a physician or other advanced-practice clinician recognized by the nurse's respective state board of nursing as having the authority to prescribe this type of interventional therapy.[6] Authorized advanced-practice clinicians may include nurse practitioners, nurse midwives, nurse anesthetists, or physician assistants. Specific information in the order must include

- Patient identification information
- Specific type of solution ordered
- Rate of administration[6]

SPEED BUMP

Specific information that must be part of an order to initiate peripheral I.V. therapy includes patient identification information, specific type of solution, and _____ .

The nurse should gather all the equipment required to gain venous access and maintain the I.V. line prior to entering the patient's room. This equipment typically includes the following:

- Prescribed I.V. solution bag hanging on an I.V. pole that is connected to I.V. tubing that is *primed,* or flushed with the solution. This I.V. setup may be connected to an I.V. pump or to extension tubing that contains additional capped access ports. Chapter 3 describes how to select and set up this equipment properly.
- Venous access device of choice (e.g., either wing-tipped needles or over-the-needle catheters).
- Single-use tourniquet.
- Povidone-iodine swab sticks and alcohol swab sticks.
- Intravenous dressing kit containing either a transparent semipermeable membrane or sterile gauze and nonallergenic tape.
- Towel to roll and place under the patient's arm, if necessary.
- Drape to place under the patient's arm.
- Disposable nonsterile gloves.[6]

PATIENT PREPARATION

Competent adult patients prescribed I.V. therapy should fully understand the intended purpose of the therapy, the anticipated length of time that the therapy will continue, and that there are some risks involved with this therapy. Patients who are prescribed I.V. therapy should understand both its associated risks and its benefits. Prescribing I.V. therapy is reserved for patients whose potential benefits outweigh the potential risks of therapy. Any adverse events that may be associated with the infusions or with the venous access devices should be discussed with patients prescribed I.V. therapy before it is begun so that they may make fully informed decisions. Even when it is the opinion of clinicians that initiating I.V. therapy is much more beneficial than harmful to the patient, decisions made by competent patients to refuse treatment must be honored as legally binding.

Most agencies require that patient informed consent be obtained prior to insertion of venous access devices. Standard 10 of the *Standards of Practice* promulgated by the Infusion Nurses Society (2006) recommends that informed consent be obtained from all competent adult patients prior to initiation of I.V. therapy.[6] In instances where the patient is either not competent to give consent or is a child or adolescent, the patient's legal representative must give consent prior to initiating I.V. therapy. Most ethicists agree that while obtaining consent of school-aged children or adolescents is not legally required prior to performing any invasive interventions on them, their assent nonetheless should be solicited.

SELECTION OF VENOUS ACCESS SITES

3 Several general conventions are followed for selection of appropriate peripheral venous access sites, including the following:

- Veins located in the upper extremities are vastly preferred as access sites.
- Distal venous access sites are tried before proximal access sites.
- Access sites that lie over points of flexion should be avoided.
- Sites that are ipsilateral to other venous access devices, arteriovenous shunts, sites of lymphatic compromise (e.g., ipsilateral-to-axillary lymph node dissection from mastectomy), and areas damaged by phlebitis and trauma should be avoided.
- If possible, veins on the nondominant arm are preferred first-line access sites rather than veins on the dominant arm.[17]

Common venous access sites include the dorsal metacarpal veins, the cephalic vein, and the basilic vein (Fig. 4-1), with the more distal sites preferred over the

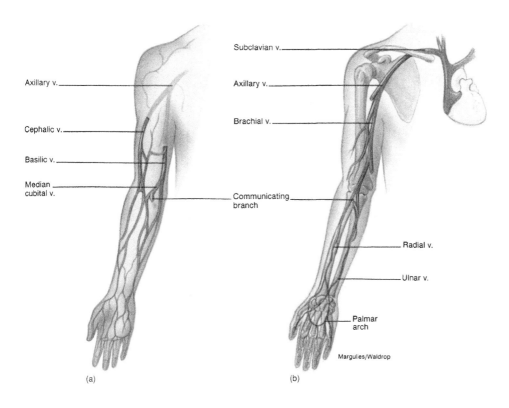

Figure 4-1 An anterior view of the veins that drain the upper right extremity. (a) Superficial veins (b) Deep veins. (Used with permission from Van De Graaff KM: *Human Anatomy*, 6th ed. New York, McGraw-Hill Higher Education, 2002:575.)

more proximal sites.[6] In instances where peripheral I.V. access must be established emergently (e.g., in cases of trauma and shock), then the larger, more readily apparent and accessible veins within the antecubital fossa are suitable first-line sites[17] (Fig. 4-2). Veins within the antecubital fossa include the median cephalic and median cubital veins.

SELECTION OF VENOUS ACCESS DEVICES

3 In general, there are two types of venous access devices that might be selected for gaining peripheral I.V. access. These include steel-winged infusion devices and over-the-needle catheters.

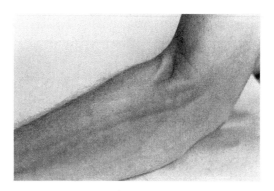

Figure 4-2   Veins of the antecubital fossa. (Used with permission from Wilson SE: *Vascular Access: Principles and Practice,* 3rd ed. St. Louis: Mosby, 1996.)

Steel-Winged Infusion Devices

Steel-winged infusion devices (sometimes referred to as *butterfly needles*) are indicated for one-time infusion of I.V. medications rather than continuous infusions of solutions or medications.[6] Although it is easier to gain I.V. access with these devices than with over-the-needle catheters, it is much more difficult to maintain I.V. access patency and stability with steel-winged infusion devices for more than 24 hours, so their use for more than a few minutes to hours is not advocated. Figure 4-3 displays a steel-winged infusion device. These devices tend to be available in a variety of gauges (G) that commonly range from 19 to 23 G. The smaller the number of the gauge, the larger is the needle bore, so 19-G devices are the largest-bored and 23-G devices are the smallest-bored steel-winged infusion devices. They are considered short peripheral devices because the length of the needle is always less than 3 inches.

Over-the-Needle Catheters

Over-the-needle catheters are the most commonly used peripheral I.V. access devices. These devices feature a needle stylet that is attached to a flash chamber. The stylet has an overlay of an over-the-needle catheter that has an attached hub device that remains external to the patient after the catheter is placed in the accessed vein.

Over-the-needle catheters are classified as **short catheters** if the catheters are 3 inches or less in length and **midline catheters** if the catheters are between 3 and 8 inches long.[6] Most catheters used for this purpose are short catheters. Midline catheters typically are reserved for use in patients who are hospitalized and require

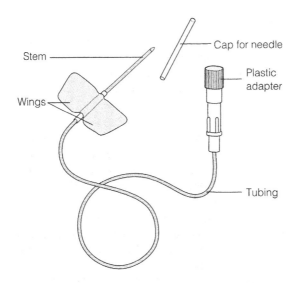

Stem

Wings

Cap for needle

Plastic adapter

Tubing

Figure 4-3 Steel-winged infusion device. (Used with permission from Berman A, Snyder SJ, Kozier B, Erb GL: *Kozier & Erb's Fundamentals of Nursing,* 8th ed. Upper Saddle River, NJ: Prentice-Hall, 2008:1460.)

frequent restarts of peripheral I.V. devices or for patients who require at least 1 week and up to 4 weeks of I.V. infusion therapy.[17] In general, it is preferred that both short and midline catheters be radiopaque.[6] These catheters are available in gauges that range from 14 to 24 G.[17]

In general, a catheter is selected so that it is of the smallest gauge and length to accomplish its intended purpose.[6] Larger-bored catheters are reserved for larger veins, which tend to be located more proximally. The larger the bore, the easier it is to infuse fluids rapidly, and the easier it is to transfuse blood components without causing the blood cells to hemolyze. In general, packed red blood cells should be infused via a venous access device that is not smaller than 18 or 20 G.[17] Figure 4-4 shows a common over-the-needle catheter device.

SPEED BUMP

In general, an I.V. access catheter is selected so that it is of the _____ gauge and length to accomplish its intended purpose.

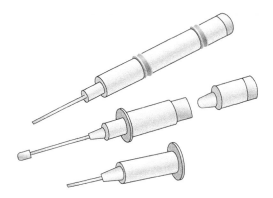

Figure 4-4 Over-the-needle infusion catheters.

GAINING VENOUS ACCESS WITH A SHORT OVER-THE-NEEDLE CATHETER

2 The nurse should explain the procedure to the patient prior to commencing the procedure to gain venous access. Any patient allergies or hypersensitivities should be ascertained, especially iodine allergies or latex allergies, so that a suitable alternate antimicrobial solution, such as chlorhexidine, may be selected or so that nonlatex gloves may be donned as needed.[17]

The patient's arm need not be washed in advance of the procedure unless is it visibly dirty.[6] The clinician should wash his or her hands vigorously with soap and water prior to beginning the procedure.[6] The I.V. bag and tubing setup that has been primed as previously described in Chapter 3 is set at the patient's bedside, and the I.V. starter kit that includes the over-the-needle catheter is opened, although the sterility of the needle stylet and catheter must be maintained. The nurse prepares several 2-inch strips of nonallergenic tape of varying widths, with some ¼ inch wide and others of 1 inch width. The preferred procedural steps for obtaining I.V. access include the following:

- A single-use tourniquet is applied to the patient's upper arm or upper portion of the forearm.[6] It is applied tightly enough to partially obstruct venous flow but not so tight as to obstruct arterial flow. The patient's arm then is dangled in a dependent position for approximately 1–2 minutes. The patient may be advised to make a fist to further encourage venous distension.[17]

- The veins are assessed so that the clinician may find a venous site suitable for access. In general, the back of the hand is assessed first, followed by sites on the ventral surface of the forearm as needed, moving from distal to proximal veins.[6] Sites are palpated to determine any areas that might feel tortuous. Tortuous sites generally are avoided.[17]

- If a site is selected and there is an excess of body hair, the hair may be clipped with scissors but not shaved. Shaving may result in dermabrasion and promote the spread of microorganisms.[17]

- After a suitable venous access site is selected, a nonsterile drape is placed under the patient's arm. The site then is cleansed with alcohol swabs in a circular motion from the center portion of the intended access site outward. This may be followed by cleansing of the site with an antimicrobial swab of povidone-iodine solution using the same motion. The site is allowed to dry for at least 30 seconds.[6]

- Nonsterile gloves are donned.[6]

- The thumb of the nondominant hand stabilizes the skin distal to the selected I.V. access site, the forefinger of the nondominant hand is fully extended under the patient's hand or arm to provide stability, and the hub of the catheter is poised in the dominant hand at a 20-degree angle to the patient's skin.[17] The catheter and needle must remain sterile and are not touched. The bevel of the needle is poised upward, away from the patient's skin (Fig. 4-5). The skin is pierced, and the needle is advanced into the vein. The clinician may feel a "popping" sensation when the vein is accessed, which is verified by noting venous blood return in the flash chamber of the device.

- The catheter angle is dropped from a 20- to a 10-degree angle flush with the patient's skin, and the catheter is advanced approximately $\frac{1}{16}$ to $\frac{1}{8}$ inch.[17]

- The needle stylet is removed gently while the catheter is advanced simultaneously into the patient's vein until only the hub is visible.

- The tourniquet is removed, and the forefinger of the nondominant hand is placed at the approximate site on the skin where the catheter tip is located, and gentle pressure is applied.

- The cap on the end of the I.V. tubing is removed and connected to the hub of the catheter.

- Intravenous solution is flushed into the catheter, and the insertion site is observed closely. Venous access is verified if there is no evidence of sudden swelling at the insertion site and if the I.V. solution can be infused briskly.[17]

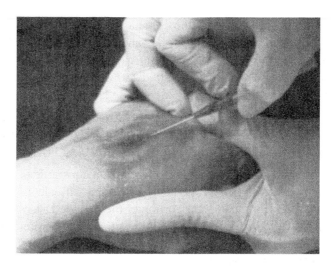

Figure 4-5   Technique for gaining vascular access using a short over-the-needle infusion catheter. (Used with permission from Hankins J, Lonsway RAW, Hedrick C, Perdue MB: *The Infusion Nurses Society: Infusion Therapy in Clinical Practice,* 2nd ed. Philadelphia: Saunders, 2001.)

- The catheter is stabilized with chevron taping, and the I.V. dressing is applied per agency or hospital policy. If the dressing chosen is a sterile gauze dressing, all sides of the gauze must be taped. If a transparent semipermeable membrane is chosen, the I.V. access site must remain visible.[5]

- The date and time of access, gauge and length of catheter inserted, and initials of nurse who started the infusion are written in ink on the dressing label.[6]

- The procedure is documented appropriately in the patient's record.[6]

GAINING VENOUS ACCESS WITH A MIDLINE OVER-THE-NEEDLE CATHETER

2   A nurse who is tasked with gaining venous access with a midline over-the-needle catheter first must demonstrate significant competency in gaining venous access using a short over-the-needle catheter.[17] The recommended procedural steps for obtaining midline I.V. access are similar to those described for short I.V. access with the following differences:

- Veins in the antecubital fossa are used for this type of venous access.[6]

- The procedure requires sterile gloves and sterile drapes.[6]

- Cleansing of the site should be done over a greater skin surface area with alcohol and then povidone-iodine swabs covering a circular area that is approximately 4 inches in diameter.[6]
- Then 0.9% normal saline (NS) is used intermittently as a flush solution of choice as the catheter is advanced to the hub.[6]

GAINING VENOUS ACCESS WITH A STEEL-WINGED INFUSION DEVICE

2 Gaining venous access with a steel-winged infusion device generally does not require more competency or experience than required to gain venous access using a short over-the-needle catheter. Indeed, some clinicians find that gaining venous access with these butterfly devices is easier because there is no catheter to thread into the vein once access is gained. However, as noted previously, maintaining continued access for more than a few hours is difficult, so indications for using these devices are limited.

Prior to initiating I.V. access with a steel-winged infusion device, the device must be prepared as follows:

- The tip and needle portion of the device must remain sterile at all times.
- A 3-, 5-, or 10-mL syringe is filled with a few milliliters of sterile 0.9% NS.
- The syringe filled with 0.9% NS is connected to the Luer-lock device at the distal end of the steel-winged infusion device.
- The line and needle of the butterfly device are flushed with some of the 0.9% NS solution, preserving at least 2–3 mL in the syringe.

After this preparatory procedure is complete, venous access may be initiated. The veins selected for access mirror the selection approach described for short over-the-needle catheters. The procedure for initiating venous access is also similar to that described for short over-the-needle catheters with the following differences:

- The device is held in the nurse's dominant hand with the bevel of the needle pointing upward (i.e., away from the patient's skin). The nurse maintains sterility of the needle by holding the wings of the device pinched between the thumb and forefinger of the dominant hand.
- Once a "popping" sensation occurs, or once there is blood flashback in the proximal end of the tubing, the device is held securely in place, and placement verification is made by aspirating more blood into the syringe. If this is difficult to accomplish, the device needs to be manipulated further.

- If blood can be aspirated readily into the syringe, then some 0.9% NS is injected into the site. If the solution can be infused readily, then the device is secured.

- Dressing methods are similar to those described for a short over-the-line catheter with the addition of tape on the wings of the device.

- The syringe is removed, the end of the device is connected to the I.V. administration setup, and the prescribed solution may infuse at the desired rate.

SECURING VENOUS ACCESS DEVICE PLACEMENT 4

I.V. Access-Site Dressing

A sterile occlusive dressing should be applied and then maintained over the I.V. access site. These dressings should be changed whenever they become soiled and at periodic intervals per agency or hospital protocols.[6] If a sterile gauze dressing is used, it should be changed at least every 48 hours. If a transparent semipermeable membrane is placed over a gauze dressing, then that dressing must be viewed as a gauze type of dressing and changed every 48 hours.[6] In general, I.V. access-site dressings that use only a transparent semipermeable membrane need to be changed only when soiled, when the membrane becomes unstable or loose, or when it is time to rotate and change the I.V. access site.[6]

Cleaning of the I.V. access site typically is done as per agency or hospital policy. Most policies specify that the site is cleansed with alcohol swabs in a circular motion from the access site outward, followed by cleansing with antimicrobial swabs such as povidone-iodine again in a circular motion from the access site outward. The site is air-dried before the catheter is stabilized once again with tape and a dressing.[6]

5 Whenever an I.V. access-site dressing is changed, a label that includes the length and gauge of the catheter, the date and time that the dressing was changed, and the initials of the person who performed the dressing change should be placed over the dressing on a site that does not obstruct visualizing the I.V. access site if a transparent semipermeable membrane is used.

Arm Board

Single-use arm boards may be indicated if the I.V. access site is at or near a point of flexion. If an arm board is used, it should not obstruct viewing the I.V. access-site dressing. Arm boards should not be used as restraint devices. Their placement and appropriate periodic assessment data should be noted in the patient's record.[6]

VENOUS ACCESS DEVICE ADVERSE EVENTS

Any time that an invasive procedure is performed and a foreign object or device is inserted, there are inherent risks. It was noted earlier that the benefits of I.V. therapy must outweigh its risks before it is prescribed for any patient. However, this does not imply that initiating I.V. therapy negates inherent risks. The risks of infusing solutions may include circulatory overload, electrolyte disturbances, and allergic reactions, to name a few. There are also risks associated with the use of peripheral venous access devices.

Risks associated with venous access devices may include the following:

- Access device displacement or "drift"

- Infiltration

- Access device contamination

- Phlebitis

- Thrombosis

The nurse must monitor carefully for evidence of any of these adverse events in patients who are recipients of peripheral I.V. therapy. Access device drift may occur because peripheral access devices are not commonly sutured into place but tend to be secured in place only with tape and dressings. To prevent displacement from occurring, it is important to use access sites on parts of the body that are manipulated infrequently, such as the nondominant arm, and not over joints. Nonetheless, even in the best of circumstances, these devices can drift, and a portion of the catheter then may become visible outside the access site. When this occurs, the site is considered violated, and the device is more likely to become contaminated. In addition, site infiltration is more likely to occur, which means that the vein at the accessed site is damaged, causing seepage of infused solution into the surrounding tissues. Infiltration typically is evidenced by redness, swelling, tenderness, and a cool sensation at the venous access site.

Access devices may become contaminated and then serve as wicks for blood-borne pathogens. This occurs most commonly if the dressing becomes soiled or wet or if the I.V. administration line setup becomes disconnected and contaminated. Contamination of the device may result in sepsis that is evidenced systemically with fever (or a low temperature in patients who are immunosuppressed), chills, rigors, and leukocytosis with an increase in bands on the white blood cell count differential. Contamination of the device may not necessarily cause a systemic infection but rather may cause a localized infection, evidenced by phlebitis or inflammation at the venous access site. This may be evidenced by redness, swelling, and pain on palpation of the access site. A palpable cord may be felt at the site, and purulent drainage may be noted. Manifestations of thrombosis tend to mirror those of phlebitis, but the underlying cause is different. When thrombosis occurs, a clot has formed at the access site. This is caused most commonly by an interruption in delivery of the I.V. solution or by improperly flushing the I.V. access device between the delivery of intermittent and bolus infusions.

Nursing strategies aimed at preventing and treating these adverse events are discussed in further detail in Chapter 6.

Changing I.V. Systems

CHANGING ADMINISTRATION SETS

5 In general, administration sets for peripheral I.V. lines should be changed no more frequently that every 72 hours or whenever it is suspected that the system has become contaminated. Whenever administration sets are changed, the entire system should be changed at the same time, including I.V. administration container and I.V. lines, including any extension tubing.[6] Some agencies and hospitals have policies that dictate that a label is attached to the I.V. administration set tubing that indicates the date and time that the administration set was last changed and the initials of the nurse who changed the set. Whenever an I.V. access site is rotated, meaning that use of one site is discontinued and a new I.V. site is accessed for continuance of infusion therapy, then the I.V. administration set should be changed completely.[6]

CONVERTING TO A LOCK DEVICE

A continuously infusing peripheral I.V. administration setup may be changed to an intermittently used capped I.V. access site referred to as a *lock device*. These lock devices are also called **saline locks** because saline (i.e., 0.9% NS) typically is the flush solution of choice, and saline remains instilled in these locks between use to keep the system patent. Figure 4-6 shows a saline lock. These devices are sometimes referred to as *heparin locks,* although heparinized solution is rarely infused into these devices as it had been in years past. It used to be thought that infused heparinized solution would be superior to saline in keeping these I.V. access devices patent, but this has been found not to be true, and there are also increased risks associated with the use of heparin that include heparin-induced thrombocytopenia (HIT). Saline locks typically are indicated for a patient who requires short-term intermittent I.V. infusions of medications.[17]

A change from a continuous I.V. administration set to a saline lock requires an order by a physician or an advanced-practice clinician with prescriptive authority.

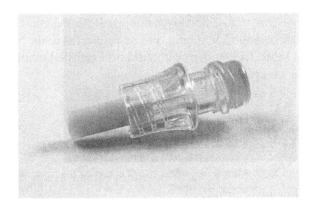

Figure 4-6   A saline lock. (Used with permission from Berman A, Snyder SJ, Kozier B, Erb GL: *Kozier & Erb's Fundamentals of Nursing*, 8th ed. Upper Saddle River, NJ: Prentice-Hall, 2008:882.)

When this order is verified as appropriate, the nurse then prepares the patient by explaining the nature of the procedure. The nurse thoroughly washes his or her hands and gathers the appropriate equipment, including an I.V. dressing kit, nonallergenic tape, and a lock device, and places these at the patient's bedside table. The lock device is flushed with sterile saline and then capped. A 3- or 5-mL syringe that is filled with sterile saline is attached to the access port of the saline lock. If the patient's I.V. access site is located near a point of flexion, then a short extension tube may be attached to the end of the saline lock and is also flushed with saline.[17]

After the appropriate equipment is gathered and the procedure is explained to the patient, a nonsterile drape is placed under the patient's hand or arm where the I.V. access site is located. The I.V. clamp is rolled shut, and if an I.V. pump is used, it is shut off after the solution infused is noted in the patient's record. Nonsterile gloves are donned, and the I.V. access-site dressing is carefully removed. After all tape is removed, the nurse places the forefinger of the nondominant hand over a site on the skin that is approximately proximal to the catheter tip and applies gentle pressure. The I.V. tubing is disconnected from the hub of the I.V. access device catheter, the cap from the saline lock or the short extension tube is removed, and the open end of the saline lock or extension tube is connected to the hub of the I.V. access device. The forefinger that had been applying gentle pressure is removed from the patient's skin, and saline is infused slowly from the prefilled syringe attached to the saline lock. The I.V. access site is observed closely for any signs of infiltration. If there are none, then the site is dressed as described earlier.

There may be times when a saline lock must be placed into a new I.V. access site. In such instances, the procedures used mimics those described in the section

"Gaining Venous Access with a Short Over-the-Needle Catheter." The key difference is that at the point where the I.V. tubing is to be connected to the hub of the venous access device, the saline lock with or without short extension tubing is connected to the hub instead, as described in this section.

Discontinuing I.V. Therapy

5 Intravenous access devices must be removed and a new access site found whenever the following occur:

- The catheter has drifted, and a portion of the catheter is visible outside the patient's skin.[6]
- The catheter has become contaminated or it is suspected that the site has become infected, which may be evidenced by redness, heat, and swelling at the I.V. access site with or without red streaks.[6]
- The catheter has infiltrated into surrounding nonvascular structures, and the site is no longer patent, as evidenced by swelling, redness, and tenderness at the site without appreciable infusion of the I.V. solution.[6]
- Thrombosis or phlebitis is suspected at the I.V. access site, which may be evidenced by redness, swelling, and pain on palpation.[6]

Intravenous access may be discontinued with an order by the patient's physician or advanced-practice clinician with prescriptive authority.[6] When this order is verified as appropriate, the nurse then prepares the patient by explaining the nature of the procedure. A nonsterile drape is placed under the patient's hand or arm where the I.V. access site is located. The nurse washes his or her hands thoroughly and has an appropriate dressing setup ready on the patient's bedside table that may include nonallergenic tape and a gauze dressing. The I.V. clamp is rolled shut, and if an I.V. pump is used, it is shut off after the solution infused is noted in the patient's record. Nonsterile gloves are donned, and the I.V. access site dressing is removed carefully. After all tape is removed, the nurse places the forefinger of the nondominant hand over a site on the skin that is approximately proximal to the catheter tip and applies gentle pressure. The sterile gauze dressing is placed loosely over the I.V. access site, and the catheter is slowly removed in one motion, pulling until it is completely removed. The gauze dressing then is applied firmly over the I.V. access site until bleeding has stopped and is taped in place with nonallergenic tape. The site is assessed in 24 hours for any evidence of infection or thrombophlebitis; if there is none, and if healing of the site has commenced, the site then may be left open to air.

Summary

Peripheral I.V. therapy is commonly indicated to treat or prevent disruption in fluid and electrolyte balance, to replace or supplement blood components, and to administer medications. A number of I.V. access devices may be chosen to gain access, although short over-the-needle catheters are indicated most commonly. In general, a venous access catheter is selected so that it is of the smallest gauge and length to accomplish its intended purpose. Peripheral I.V. lines must be maintained appropriately so that system sterility and patency are ensured.

Quiz

1. Which of the following is the *least* common indication for initiating peripheral I.V. therapy?

    (a) To treat and prevent fluid and electrolyte disturbances

    (b) To replace or supplement blood components

    (c) To administer medications

    (d) To provide parenteral nutrition

2. Which of the following might be a preferred peripheral venous access site?

    (a) A vein that lies over a point of flexion

    (b) A nontortuous metacarpal vein on a nondominant hand

    (c) A median cephalic vein that is ipsilateral to the side where the patient had a previous axillary lymph node dissection

    (d) A vein in the nondominant leg

3. Which of the following I.V. infusion devices is indicated for one-time-only administration of a medication?

    (a) A steel winged-tipped infusion device

    (b) A short over-the-needle catheter

    (c) A midline over-the-needle catheter

    (d) A heparin lock device

4. An I.V. administration set should be changed

    (a) every 24 hours.

    (b) every 48 hours.

(c) whenever the system is contaminated.

(d) every other time a new I.V. access site is initiated.

5. Which part of the over-the-needle catheter must remain sterile?

(a) The hub

(b) The flash chamber

(c) The catheter

(d) The connecting tubing

6. Transparent semipermeable membrane I.V. dressings should be changed

(a) every 48 hours.

(b) every 72 hours.

(c) whenever they are soiled.

(d) as per protocol for transparent semipermeable membrane dressings when a gauze dressing lies underneath the membrane.

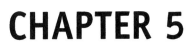

CHAPTER 5

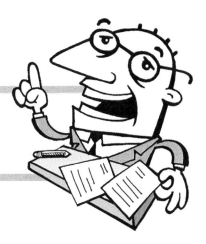

Central Intravenous Therapy

Learning Objectives

After completing this chapter, the learner will

1. Discuss indications for delivering intravenous (I.V.) therapy by the central route.

2. Describe advantages and disadvantages to selecting common peripheral and central access sites when central venous access is indicated.

3. Compare and contrast indications for peripherally inserted central catheters, tunneled central venous catheters, percutaneous central venous catheters, and implanted ports.

4 Compare and contrast I.V. delivery setup features of peripherally inserted central catheters, tunneled central venous catheters, percutaneous central venous catheters, and implanted ports.

5 Compare and contrast common adverse events associated with use of peripherally inserted central catheters, tunneled central venous catheters, percutaneous central venous catheters, and implanted ports.

Key Terms

Infiltrate   Phlebitis
Vesicants   Valsalva maneuver

Indications for Central Intravenous (I.V.) Therapy

1 Indications for central I.V. therapy mirror those for peripheral I.V. therapy. That is, central I.V. therapy is indicated to prevent or treat disturbances in fluid and electrolyte balance, to replace or supplement blood components, to administer medications, or to provide a parenteral route for delivery of nutrients.

In general, administering any solution by the central I.V. route carries greater risk than administering a solution peripherally. There is a greater risk for iatrogenically induced sepsis, thrombosis, and air embolism for patients who have central I.V. lines than for those who have peripheral I.V. lines. Patients who have centrally inserted I.V. lines are also at increased risk for pneumothorax and hemothorax, which can occur during the time of catheter insertion. Therefore, there are specific indications for initiating and maintaining central I.V. therapy. A general rule of thumb is that the benefits must outweigh the risks whenever central I.V. therapy is prescribed.

Peripheral I.V. lines do not tend to maintain their patency after 48–72 hours, and they **infiltrate**, meaning that the vessels become fragile and lose their integrity. The I.V. solution then infuses into the surrounding tissues rather than into the vessel.[6] Patients scheduled to be maintained on I.V. therapy for several days, weeks, or months must have stable I.V. access. If peripheral I.V. venous access sites were to be rotated repeatedly every 2–3 days, finding suitable healthy access sites quickly would become difficult. Therefore, patients who are expected to require I.V. therapy for more than 7 days are candidates for central I.V. therapy.[17]

SPEED BUMP

_____ *occurs when veins that are accessed by I.V. delivery devices lose their integrity, and I.V. solution infuses into surrounding tissues.*

A great many pharmacologic agents are administered intravenously that are vesicants. **Vesicants** are agents that may cause blistering.[6] Thus vesicants can cause significant venous irritation that typically is more pronounced in smaller vessels. Vesicants may cause inflammatory changes in smaller vessels, a condition referred to as **phlebitis**.[6] Phlebitis causes not only pain and discomfort for the patient, but it also can compromise the integrity of venous access and patency of I.V. flow. There are many pharmacologic agents that are vesicants, but some significant general categories include chemotherapeutic agents and vasopressors (e.g., dopamine).

The delivery of total parenteral nutrient solutions via the peripheral route also can cause phlebitis. Therefore, another common indication to initiate central I.V. therapy in a patient is to deliver nutritionally complete parenteral nutrition. Nutritional solutions delivered by the central I.V. route may include total parenteral nutrition (TPN), intravenous fat emulsions (IVFEs), and total nutrient admixtures (TNAs), which are discussed in more detail in Chapter 10.

Central Venous Access Routes

2 There are several routes by which central veins might be accessed by I.V. lines, which most commonly use specially designed I.V. catheters. It is possible to thread a lengthy I.V. catheter by a peripheral access site into a central vein. These types of peripherally accessed central catheters are referred to as *peripherally inserted central catheters* (PICCs).[6] Insertion of PICCs does not carry the risks of hemothorax or pneumothorax that might occur when central sites are used for central venous access. Other venous access sites are central and commonly include the subclavian vein and internal jugular vein and less commonly the external jugular vein and femoral vein.[6] The external jugular vein tends to be a less stable site than the internal jugular vein or the subclavian vein and therefore is not a preferred first-line large access vessel. The femoral access route tends to carry greater risks for septicemia given its proximity to the anus and urethral orifice and therefore is also not as preferable a first-line vessel as the internal jugular vein and subclavian vein. Central I.V. lines that are accessed by central sites may include tunneled central venous catheters, percutaneous central venous catheters, and implanted ports. Each of these will be discussed in the following sections.

SPEED BUMP

The _____ vein and the _____ vein are both preferred first-line venous access sites for insertion of central venous catheters.

PATIENT PREPARATION

Many state regulations and laws require that patient informed consent must be obtained prior to initiating a central I.V. line, including a PICC line. If this is the case, the nurse must ensure that this has been obtained. Competent adult patients prescribed central I.V. therapy should fully understand the intended purpose of the therapy, the anticipated length of time that the therapy will continue, and the risks associated with this therapy. Prescribing central I.V. therapy is reserved for patients whose potential benefits outweigh the potential risks of therapy. Any adverse events that may be associated with the infusions, with the venous access devices, or with the procedure used to gain central venous access should be discussed with patients prescribed central I.V. therapy before it is begun so that they may make fully informed decisions. Even when it is the opinion of clinicians that initiating I.V. therapy is much more beneficial than harmful to the patient, decisions made by competent patients to refuse treatment must be honored as legally binding.

Standard 10 of the *Standards of Practice* promulgated by the Infusion Nurses Society (2006) recommends that informed consent be obtained from all competent adult patients prior to initiation of any type of I.V. therapy.[6] In instances where the patient is either not competent to give consent or is a child or adolescent, the patient's legal representative must give consent prior to initiating central I.V. therapy. Most ethicists agree that while obtaining consent of children or adolescents is not legally required prior to performing any invasive interventions on them, their assent nonetheless should be solicited. As is true with any procedure, the nurse explains the nature of the central I.V. line insertion to the patient in advance, answers any questions the patient may have, and allays any procedurally related anxiety the patient may experience.

PERIPHERALLY INSERTED CENTRAL CATHETER

3 Peripherally inserted central catheters (PICCs) are indicated for patients who require continuous or intermittent I.V. therapy for at least 7 days. PICCs may remain in place for up to several months. **4** PICCs are inserted into veins in the antecubital fossa and are threaded until the tip of the catheter reaches the lower third of the superior vena cava, just above the junction of the right atrium.[6,17] Figure 5-1 displays the correct placement of a PICC.

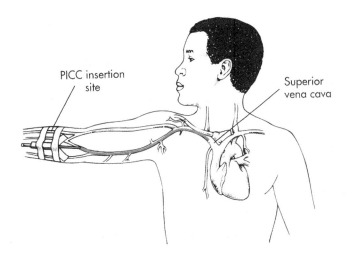

Figure 5-1 Properly inserted PICC, with tip in the superior vena cava. (Used with permission from Perry AG, Potter PA: *Clinical Nursing Skills and Techniques,* 5th ed. St. Louis: Mosby, 2002:582.)

Nurses may insert PICCs if performing this procedure is approved as within their domain of practice by their individual state boards of nursing. If this is the case, then most hospitals and health care agencies enforce specific policies that dictate the competency that a nurse must demonstrate prior to inserting a PICC line. Most agencies and hospitals require that nurses eligible to insert PICCs first must attend classes on PICC line insertion and also demonstrate sufficient psychomotor mastery of venipuncture techniques and gaining venous access on multiple patients using short and midline catheters.

The nurse must gather all appropriate equipment prior to initiating the therapy. This equipment typically includes the following:

- A catheter must be selected for insertion. **4** PICCs are available in gauge (G) sizes that range from 24 to 16 G. The smaller the number of the gauge, the larger is the diameter of the catheter. Smaller-gauged PICCs, such as 24- and 22-G catheters, may be appropriate in children and in frail elderly adults. It is difficult to transfuse blood products in a line that is smaller than 20 G, however, and this may need to be considered when selecting an appropriate PICC size.

- PICCs are also available in a variety of lengths, from 40 to 65 cm. The length of the catheter is selected based on the size of the patient. Each patient should be measured to select the appropriate length of catheter. A tape measure may be used to accomplish this. The end of the tape should be placed approximately one fingerbreadth below the patient's antecubital fossa, extended up to the shoulder, across the shoulder to the sternal notch, and then down to the third intercostal space. The length of this measurement plus 1 cm is the approximate length of catheter that should be selected.

- It is possible to trim catheters for a better fit, but the catheter must remain sterile, and therefore, the nurse must ensure that this done on a sterile field using sterile equipment.

Once the appropriate PICC is selected, other equipment that should be gathered includes the following:

- One extension tube and cap for each access port on the catheter
- A single-use tourniquet
- A PICC or central line access and dressing kit, which may contain the following:
  - Povidone-iodine swab sticks and alcohol swab sticks
  - Scissors
  - Anesthetic agent, such as 1% lidocaine or a dermal anesthetic cream (e.g., EMLA cream)
  - Several 10-mL syringes filled with sterile 0.9% normal saline (NS)
  - Several 21-G needles
  - Several 4 × 4 inch and 2 × 2 inch sterile gauze pads
  - Transparent semipermeable membrane
  - Sterile drape to place under the patient's arm and a sterile fenestrated drape to place over the patient's prepped antecubital fossa
- Towel to roll and place under the patient's arm, if necessary
- Heparinized flush solution (e.g., 100 units heparin/mL)
- Protective mask, gown, and goggles for the nurse, plus a mask for the patient
- Two pairs of disposable sterile gloves[6]

Gaining Venous Access

After the procedure has been explained to the patient, informed consent has been obtained, and the necessary equipment has been gathered, the nurse thoroughly and vigorously washes his or her hands and forearms using antiseptic soap for 60 seconds. He or she then assists the patient to a dorsal recumbent position, gently assists the patient to abduct the preferred arm (e.g., nondominant arm) to a 45- to 90-degree angle from the torso, and begins the steps to initiate venous access.

- A protective nonsterile drape is placed under the patient's arm.

- A single-use tourniquet is applied to the patient's upper arm just below the axilla.[6] It is applied tightly enough to partially obstruct venous flow but not so tight as to obstruct arterial flow. The patient's arm then is dangled in a dependent position for approximately 1–2 minutes. A roll may be placed under the patient's upper arm. The patient may be advised to make a fist to further encourage venous distension.

- The veins are assessed so that the nurse can find a venous site suitable for access. The veins that are preferred for use include the basilic, median cubital, and cephalic veins,[6] which are shown in Fig. 5-2. Sites are palpated to determine any areas that might feel tortuous. Tortuous sites generally are avoided.[17] After the site is selected, the tourniquet is released.

- If a site is selected and there is an excess of body hair, the hair may be clipped with scissors but not shaved. Shaving may result in dermabrasion and promote the spread of microorganisms.[17]

- The nurse gently places a face mask on the patient and then dons a gown, goggles, and face mask.

- A sterile field is opened, and equipment that is packed sterile is dropped onto the sterile field. This may include packets of gauze, transparent semipermeable membranes, 10-mL syringes, and sterile-packed vials of

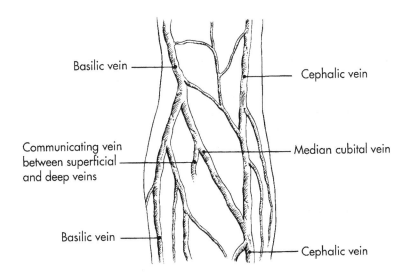

Figure 5-2   Veins in the antecubital fossa. (Used with permission from Wilson SE: *Vascular Access: Principles and Practice,* 3rd ed. St. Louis: Mosby, 1996:24.)

lidocaine and saline. Some agencies and hospitals stock ready-made central venous access kits with all the necessary equipment packed inside the sterile-packed kit.

- The nurse dons the first pair of sterile gloves and prepares the catheter on the sterile field by flushing it via all lumens with sterile saline (i.e., 0.9% NS). The extension tubes likewise are flushed and capped.

- A sterile drape is placed under the patient's arm.

- The patient's identified venous access site is prepared by cleansing it with alcohol swabs in a circular motion from the center portion of the intended access site outward to a total diameter of 10 inches. This must be repeated three to five times. This is followed by cleansing the site with an antimicrobial swab of povidone-iodine solution using the same motions. The site is allowed to dry for at least 60 seconds.[6]

- The tourniquet is reapplied, the first pair of gloves is removed, and a second pair of sterile gloves is donned.[6]

- The patient's arm is draped with a sterile fenestrated drape, leaving an opening over the intended access site.

- The site is anesthetized with an injection of 1% lidocaine or with dermal anesthetic cream.

- The selected site is accessed using the catheter's introducer needle. Once access is gained, the stylet is slowly pulled back until it is removed, and the introducer is advanced.

- The tourniquet is released.

- The catheter is advanced slowly over a period of 5–10 minutes, checking at intermittent intervals by alternately aspirating for blood return and flushing with saline. When the catheter has advanced halfway, the patient should be asked to turn his or her head toward the shoulder of the insertion site, and the introducer then is removed. The remaining length of the catheter then is advanced, and the guidewire is removed slowly.[17]

- Blood is once more aspirated from the catheter, and more saline is flushed through the system.

- The extension tube(s) of the setup that is(are) primed with saline are capped.

- The site either is secured with the manufacturer's PICC stabilization device or is sutured into place. A sterile dressing is placed over the site, which may include a sterile gauze dressing with a transparent semipermeable membrane.

- Access ports are flushed with heparinized flush solution.

- The date and time of access, gauge and length of catheter inserted, and initials of nurse who started the PICC are written in ink on the dressing label.[6]

- Catheter placement is verified with a chest x-ray prior to initiation of I.V. fluids.

- The procedure is documented appropriately in the patient's record.[6]

Maintaining Venous Access

PICC access sites do not need to be rotated unless the site appears thrombotic or it is suspected that the catheter is a source of infection. If a PICC line becomes partially dislodged, it should not be readvanced.[6] Gauze dressings should be changed every 48 hours and whenever they are loosened or soiled. Gauze dressings that have a transparent semipermeable membrane overlay are treated as if they are gauze dressings and changed every 48 hours. Dressings that use a transparent semipermeable membrane without gauze may be changed as infrequently as every 7 days as long as they remain intact and not soiled.

The equipment needed to change a PICC dressing includes the following:

- Mask

- One pair of nonsterile gloves and one pair of sterile gloves

- Alcohol swabs

- Povidone-iodine swabs

- Dressing
    - 4 × 4 sterile gauze and tape or
    - Transparent semipermeable membrane

Many manufacturer's market ready-made central I.V. line dressing kits that tend to include all the preceding supplies in a ready-to-go package.

The following steps describe a procedure that might be followed to change a PICC dressing:

- The nurse thoroughly and vigorously washes his or her hands for at least 60 seconds.

- The nature of the procedure is explained to the patient, and any questions the patient may have are answered. The patient is assisted into a dorsal recumbent position, and the patient's head is turned so that it is facing away from the PICC insertion site.

- The sterile equipment is opened using sterile technique and set aside for future use.

- The nurse applies the mask and nonsterile gloves.

- The nurse gently removes the dressing, carefully lifting it from the insertion site so as not to dislodge the catheter.
- The insertion site and catheter are inspected for any evidence of drifting, cracking, infection, or phlebitis.
- The nurse removes the nonsterile gloves and dons the sterile gloves.
- The site is cleansed with alcohol swabs from the center of the insertion site outward using a circular motion. The line then is cleansed with an alcohol swab from the insertion site to the end. If sutures are present, they are also cleansed with alcohol. The alcohol is allowed to dry.
- The site then is cleansed with povidone-iodine swabs using the same technique as described previously for cleansing with alcohol swabs.
- The site is dressed per agency or hospital policy using either a gauze dressing or a transparent semipermeable membrane. If a gauze dressing is used, the ends of the dressing must be sealed completely with tape or a transparent semipermeable membrane.
- The date and time that the dressing was changed, the gauge and length of the catheter inserted, and initials of nurse who performed the dressing change are written in ink on the dressing label.
- The procedure is documented appropriately in the patient's record.[6]

There are some activity and procedural restrictions that patients should be cautioned to adhere to preserve function of the PICC for the longest time possible. Blood pressure readings and venipunctures should not be permitted on the arm that has the PICC line. Patients must be cautioned not to get the PICC dressing wet or dirty. Dressings should be covered with a protective barrier when patients take showers so that they cannot get wet or otherwise contaminated. Activities likewise should be restricted that could either damage the catheter or cause the catheter to drift. These include lifting of objects weighing more than 10 pounds and any activities that might entail repeated use of the arm or that might cause the elbow to flex repeatedly.

CENTRAL VENOUS CATHETERS

Central I.V. catheters inserted into central venous access sites, including the subclavian vein, the internal jugular vein, the external jugular vein, and the femoral vein, are inserted either surgically or percutaneously. Central I.V. catheters that are inserted surgically are inserted in an operating room or surgical suite, and those inserted percutaneously are done at the patient's bedside or in a procedure or treatment room using sterile technique. All central I.V. catheters that use a central venous access site must be inserted by physicians or by advanced-practice clinicians such as nurse practitioners, nurse midwives, nurse anesthetists, and physician assistants who have the authority to do so by their respective state boards of medicine and nursing. Patients whose subclavian or jugular veins are accessed directly by central catheters have a heightened risk of hemothorax, pneumothorax, air embolism, thrombosis, and infection.[6]

4 Centrally inserted I.V. lines include tunneled catheters and implantable ports. Tunneled catheters are so named because they are accessed through a surgically created subcutaneous tunnel that the catheter traverses between tissue on the chest wall, typically between the sternum and a nipple, and the vein, typically the subclavian vein. Tunneled catheters maintain access-site stability longer and are associated with smaller rates of infection than nontunneled central lines.[17] These catheters feature Dacron cuffs at the wall exit site that soon is surrounded by a cuff of fibrous tissue. This fibrous tissue serves the dual functions of providing line stability and providing a barrier that is difficult for pathogens to penetrate and thus thwarts them from gaining access to the vasculature.[17]

3 Implantable ports are inserted so that patients may receive intermittent infusions of chemotherapeutic agents, blood components, and parenteral nutrients over several months. These ports also can serve as a site for withdrawal of blood specimens. Patients who have implantable ports frequently have cancer and are expected to receive numerous rounds of chemotherapy. Often these patients also must submit blood specimens so that results from laboratory analyses can be used to guide therapy. Blood specimens may be withdrawn readily from the port, saving sick patients from multiple venipunctures. So that the membranes on these ports are not ruptured, a special noncoring needle called a *Huber needle* is used. Figure 5-3 shows

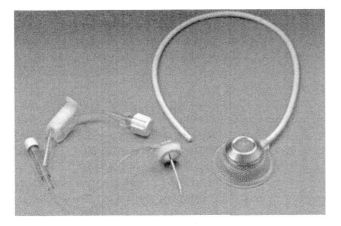

Figure 5-3   Implantable venous access device with a Huber needle and tubing. (From Berman A, Snyder SJ, Kozier B, Erb GL: *Kozier & Erb's Fundamentals of Nursing,* 8*th* ed. Upper Saddle River, NJ: Prentice-Hall, 2008:1458.)

a typical implantable port with a Huber needle. These devices are inserted subcutaneously on the chest wall, and the subclavian vein is the most commonly selected venous access site.

Percutaneously inserted central catheters may be inserted at the bedside. These types of central I.V. lines must be inserted by a physician or by an advanced-practice clinician, as described previously. The nurse typically assists during these sterile procedures, and the equipment setup is similar to that used for insertion of a PICC, as described earlier. The accurate placement of these lines also must be verified by x-rays before solutions can be infused safely. Figure 5-4 presents two illustrations of percutaneously inserted central catheters.

4 There are many different types of central venous catheter products that can be selected for any given patient. Some catheters have multiple access ports or lumens that may be used for infusing multiple types of solutions. Figure 5-5 shows two common types of catheters, one with a single lumen and another with a triple lumen.

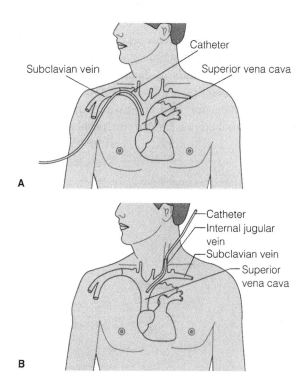

Figure 5-4 Central venous catheters. *A.* Subclavian central venous catheter. *B.* Internal jugular central venous catheter. (Used with permission from Berman A, Snyder SJ, Kozier B, Erb GL: *Kozier & Erb's Fundamentals of Nursing,* 8th ed. Upper Saddle River, NJ: Prentice-Hall, 2008:1457.)

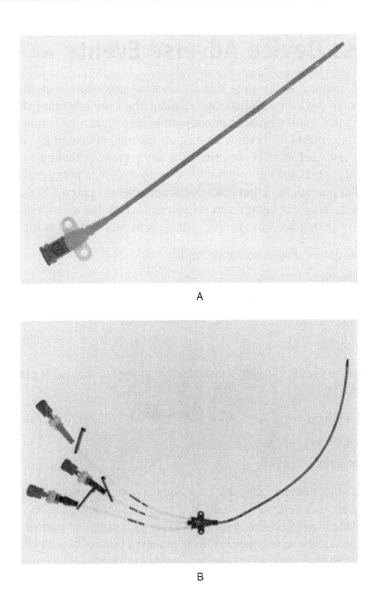

A

B

Figure 5-5   Central venous catheters. *A.* Single-lumen. *B.* Triple-lumen catheter. (From Wilson SE: *Vascular Access: Principles and Practice,* 3rd ed. St. Louis: Mosby, 1996:71.)

Patients with central I.V. lines must maintain sterile dressings over their access sites that are the same types of dressings that cover PICC insertion sites. The schedule and technique for changing these dressings are virtually the same as those described previously for changing PICC insertion-site dressings.

Venous Access Device Adverse Events 5

As noted in Chapter 4, any time that an invasive procedure is performed and a foreign object or device is inserted into a patient, there are inherent risks. The same rule of thumb that guides whether or not peripheral I.V. therapy is indicated guides indications for central I.V. therapy. That is, the benefits of central I.V. therapy must outweigh its risks before it is prescribed for any patient. Although some risks are less commonly associated with central I.V. therapy than with peripheral I.V. therapy, there are other potentially lethal risks that are unique to central I.V. therapy. Risks associated with the use of central venous access devices that mirror risks associated with the use of peripheral venous access devices include the following:

- Access device displacement or "drift"
- Infiltration
- Access device contamination
- Phlebitis
- Thrombosis

Other adverse events that may occur that are unique to the use of central venous access devices include

- Air embolism
- Pneumothorax
- Hemothorax

The nurse must monitor carefully for evidence of any of these adverse events in patients who are recipients of central I.V. therapy. In particular, access device drift may occur, which can become visually evident by noting that part of the catheter has drifted outside the access site. This occurs less commonly with central venous access devices that are sutured in place and least commonly with the use of tunneled catheters or implantable ports. The most common central venous access devices that become displaced in this fashion are PICCs that are not sutured in place, especially if they are placed in the dominant arm. When drift occurs, the site is considered violated, and the device is more likely to become contaminated. In addition, site infiltration is more likely to occur, which means that the vein at the site is damaged, causing seepage of infused solution into the surrounding tissues. Infiltration typically is evidenced by redness, swelling, tenderness, and a cool sensation at the venous access site. In general, however, infiltration occurs much less commonly when a central venous access device is used than when a peripheral venous access device is used.

Access devices may become contaminated and then serve as wicks for blood-borne pathogens. This occurs most commonly if the dressing becomes soiled or wet or if the I.V. administration line setup becomes disconnected and contaminated. Contamination of the device may result in sepsis that is evidenced systemically by fever (or a low temperature in patients who are immunosuppressed), chills, rigor, and leukocytosis with an increase in bands on the white blood count differential. Device-associated sepsis occurs more commonly with use of central access routes than with peripheral access routes. Contamination of the device also may be implicated in causing phlebitis, which may be evidenced by redness, swelling, and pain on palpation of the access site. A palpable cord may be felt at the site, and purulent drainage may be noted.

Manifestations of thrombosis tend to mirror those of phlebitis, but the underlying cause is different. When thrombosis occurs, a clot has formed at the access site. This is caused most commonly by an interruption in delivery of I.V. solution or by improperly flushing the I.V. access device between the delivery of intermittent or bolus infusions. In general, central venous access devices are more prone to forming thrombi than are peripheral venous access devices. Whereas thrombus formation may not cause problematic emboli when they are located in peripheral vessels, they can become lethal pulmonary emboli if they are present in central vessels.

Air emboli may form if air is introduced into a central vessel, from air bubbles that either are infused with the I.V. infusion or result from disconnection of the I.V. administration line set. These air emboli can cause the same lethal consequences as thrombi that dislodge and become clotted emboli and cause pulmonary embolism, respiratory distress, and possibly respiratory failure.

Patients with centrally accessed central I.V. lines are at risk for the potentially lethal adverse events of pneumothorax and hemothorax during the time that the line is inserted. These adverse events may be manifested by dyspnea, respiratory distress, hypoxemia, and eventual cardiopulmonary failure.

Nursing strategies aimed at preventing and treating these adverse events are discussed in further detail in Chapter 6.

Discontinuing Central I.V. Therapy

Central I.V. catheters should be removed whenever it is suspected that they are contaminated or a source of infection, whenever they are damaged, and whenever it is determined by the patient's physician that I.V. therapy is no longer warranted. PICCs and nontunneled central catheters may be discontinued by a nurse, whereas tunneled central catheters and implanted ports must be discontinued surgically.[6]

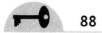

The nurse tasked with removing a PICC line or a nontunneled central I.V. line should be mindful that air embolism formation is the most serious adverse event that might occur during this procedure. Prior to removing either one of these catheters, the nurse explains the procedure to the patient, answers any questions that the patient may have, and allays any anxiety. Supplies gathered include the following:

- A mask and nonsterile gloves
- A suture removal kit
- Several sterile 4 × 4 inch gauze pads and tape
- Antibiotic ointment

General procedural guidelines for removal of a PICC or a nontunneled central catheter include the following:

- The I.V. pump is turned off or the I.V. line is clamped if solution is infusing continuously into the I.V. delivery system.
- The patient is assisted to the dorsal recumbent position and asked to turn his or her head away from the dressing site. The nurse dons a mask and nonsterile gloves and carefully removes the dressing.
- Any sutures are removed with the scissors and tweezers in the suture removal kit.
- The nurse holds a sterile gauze pad over the access site and instructs the patient to perform the **Valsalva maneuver** to prevent an air embolus from entering the open venous access site. This means that the patient is instructed to forcefully exhale against the closed glottis. The line then is gently removed.
- If resistance is met during catheter removal, the nurse does not continue to pull but dresses the exposed catheter with a sterile dressing and notifies the physician promptly. If the catheter can be removed without resistance, it is completely pulled out, antibiotic ointment is applied over the site, and a sterile occlusive dressing is placed firmly over the access site.
- The catheter is examined to ensure that there is no evidence of damage. If there is any cracking or other notable damage, this is promptly reported to the manufacturer, typically through the hospital or health care agency's risk management office.
- The removal procedure is documented in the patient's record.
- The site is reexamined every 24 hours to determine if healing is occurring. Once the site has apparently epithelialized, it may be left open to air.[6]

Summary

Central I.V. lines may be indicated for patients who are prescribed I.V. therapy that is anticipated to last for more than 7 days. Key risks associated with insertion and maintenance of many of these devices include air embolism, thrombosis, infection, pneumothorax, and hemothorax. Selection of the type of central access device is predicated on the type of therapy that is prescribed for the patient. In general, the I.V. access route and method of delivery are determined based on weighing the risks and benefits of therapy.

Quiz

1. Which of the following central I.V. lines carries the lowest risk of access-associated pneumothorax?

    (a) PICC

    (b) Tunneled catheter

    (c) Implantable port

    (d) Percutaneously inserted subclavian line

2. Identify the vein that could be selected as an access site for a PICC line?

    (a) Basilic

    (b) Subclavian

    (c) External jugular

    (d) Femoral

3. Identify the vein that provides the best access site for a centrally inserted central I.V. line.

    (a) Basilic

    (b) Subclavian

    (c) External jugular

    (d) Femoral

4. Which of the following adverse events or complications is *a less common occurrence* with central I.V. lines than with peripheral I.V. lines?

    (a) Pneumothorax

    (b) Air embolism

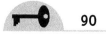

    (c) Infection

    (d) Infiltration

5. Which of the following adverse events or complications is the most worrisome in patients who are having their central I.V. lines discontinued?

    (a) Pneumothorax

    (b) Air embolism

    (c) Infection

    (d) Infiltration

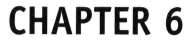

CHAPTER 6

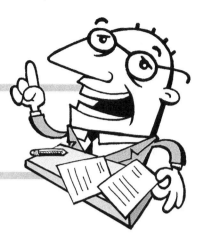

Intravenous Therapy and the Nursing Process

Learning Objectives

After completing this chapter, the learner will

1. Understand the applicability of the nursing process for patients who are prescribed intravenous (I.V.) therapy.

2. Identify the interplay between the taxonomies of the North American Nursing Diagnosis Association (NANDA), the Nursing Outcomes Classification (NOC), and the Nursing Interventions Classification (NIC).

3. Recognize common actual and potential nursing diagnoses for patients who are prescribed I.V. therapy.

4. Plan appropriate care for a patient receiving I.V. therapy based on actual and potential nursing diagnoses.

Key Terms

Nursing process

North American Nursing Diagnosis
Association (NANDA)

Nursing Outcomes Classification (NOC)

Nursing Interventions Classification (NIC)

Review of the Nursing Process

1 The **nursing process** is the scientific reasoning used by professional nurses when they assess, diagnose, plan, intervene, and evaluate plans of care for patients, families, communities, and populations who have health concerns. Nurses who provide care to patients who are prescribed intravenous (I.V.) therapy must be attuned to focusing their clinical reasoning skills on the actual and potential nursing diagnoses that are experienced most commonly by patients receiving I.V. therapy. These diagnoses can form the framework for designing specific plans of care for these patients. **2** This chapter focuses on those specific **North American Nursing Diagnosis Association (NANDA)** nursing diagnoses that are particularly salient for patients who are prescribed I.V. therapy. NANDA compiles a professionally agreed-on taxonomy of actual and potential nursing diagnoses.[18]

SPEED BUMP

_____ *is the professional nursing organization that compiles a professionally agreed-on taxonomy of actual and potential nursing diagnoses.*

The nursing diagnoses that are highlighted in this chapter may or may not apply to each and every patient who receives I.V. therapy. In addition, this list of diagnoses is generic and does not take into account individual patient characteristics; therefore, it is certainly not an exhaustive list. It merely provides a common framework so that general plans of care that are aimed at treating and preventing clinical sequelae common to patients receiving I.V. therapy can be further identified and discussed. The framework for the plans of care uses additional taxonomic terms disseminated by the **Nursing Outcomes Classification (NOC)** and the **Nursing Interventions Classification (NIC)**, respectively. Taxonomic terms used by NOC and NIC are promulgated by the Center for Nursing Classification at the University of Iowa.[19]

SPEED BUMP

_____ is a taxonomic classification system for nursing outcomes that is promulgated by the Center for Nursing Classification at the University of Iowa.

Common Nursing Diagnoses for Patients Receiving I.V. Therapy

3 Nursing diagnoses that are commonly applicable for patients receiving I.V. therapy include

- Deficient fluid volume
- Risk for infection
- Risk for injury
- Risk for disuse syndrome
- Anxiety
- Deficient knowledge

General plans of care for patients receiving I.V. therapy that might be appropriately derived from each of these nursing diagnoses will be discussed in the following sections.

DEFICIENT FLUID VOLUME

4 Deficient fluid volume that is related to either extracellular or intracellular fluid loss is a common reason that patients are prescribed I.V. therapy. These patients must be monitored continuously to ensure that they are exhibiting a positive clinical response to I.V. therapy.

Key assessment parameters that a nurse might find when this nursing diagnosis is made may include any or all of the following:

Subjective

- Weakness
- Thirst

Objective

- Decreased skin turgor
- Dry mucus membranes
- Increased heart rate
- Decreased blood pressure
- Decreased pulse pressure
- Decreased capillary refill
- Change in mental status or level of orientation
- Decreased urine output
- Increased urine specific gravity
- Elevated hemoglobin and hematocrit
- Sudden weight loss[18]

Similar types of nursing diagnoses that also may be applicable include the following:

- Risk for deficient fluid volume
- Risk for imbalanced fluid volume[18]

Patient risk factors for deficient fluid volume that can prompt the physician or advanced-practice clinician with prescriptive authority (e.g., nurse practitioner, nurse midwife, nurse anesthetist, and physician assistant) to prescribe I.V. therapy might include the following:

- Any condition causing a hypermetabolic state (e.g., severe sepsis, severe burns, or multiple trauma)
- Use of medications that can cause dehydration (e.g., diuretics)
- Loss of fluids through placement of invasive devises (e.g., nasogastric tubes)
- Loss of fluids through the gastrointestinal tract from illness (e.g., vomiting and diarrhea)
- Lack of ability to self-hydrate because of either cognitive deficiencies (e.g., dementia or delirium) or physical immobility[18]

Patients at risk for an imbalance in their fluid volume status who likewise might be prescribed I.V. therapy include those scheduled for major surgical procedures[18] (e.g., patients whose surgical procedures take longer than 30 minutes). In addition, patients receiving I.V. therapy because of deficiencies in fluid volume are at risk for the complication of excess fluid volume if their I.V. fluids are administered overzealously, and they must be monitored for clinical manifestations suggestive of fluid volume overload.

Expected outcomes for patients receiving I.V. therapy who are diagnosed with deficient fluid volume or who are diagnosed as at risk for deficient fluid volume or imbalanced fluid volume include the following:

- The patient will achieve electrolyte and acid–base balance.
- The patient will achieve fluid balance.
- The patient will be adequately hydrated.[19]

Nursing interventions that may be appropriate to ensure that patients receiving I.V. therapy achieve these expected outcomes may include the following:

- Key subjective and objective assessment parameters that were identified previously for improvement, stabilization, or deterioration in the patient's fluid volume status are reassessed continuously.
- The patient's intake and output are assessed and documented on a daily basis.
- The patient's daily weight is assessed and documented.
- The patient's I.V. therapy administration setup is maintained using the prescribed solution, and the solution is delivered at the prescribed rate.
- The patient's vital signs are monitored at prescribed intervals.
- Key laboratory findings are assessed to determine whether the patient's fluid volume status has improved, stabilized, or deteriorated. These may include a complete blood count (CBC), serum chemistries, and urinalysis (UA).
- The effects of prescribed medications that might further contribute to or exacerbate fluid volume loss (e.g., diuretics) are monitored.
- The effects of prescribed therapies that might further contribute to or exacerbate fluid volume loss (e.g., nasogastric tubes) are monitored.[19]

RISK FOR INFECTION

4 A patient who has any type of invasive procedure is at risk for infection.[18] Patients who are receiving I.V. therapy have an invasive procedure performed that results in the placement of a venous access device that can serve as a wick for

transmission of pathogens to the patient. Patients receiving I.V. therapy who are particularly at heightened risk for infection include

- Patients with contaminated I.V. dressings, I.V. access sites, and I.V. solutions or delivery systems.
- Patients who have multiple concomitant chronic illnesses.
- Patients who are immunosuppressed (e.g., patients with AIDS, active neoplasms, or receiving corticosteroids).
- Patients who are malnourished.[18]

The expected outcome for patients receiving I.V. therapy is that they remain free from infection.[19] Nursing interventions that help to ensure this include the following:

- Asepsis is maintained in the I.V. delivery system by periodically changing the delivery setup while maintaining sterility of the solution and interconnections as per agency or hospital protocol, as specified in Chapter 3.
- The I.V. dressing is changed periodically as per guidelines specified in Chapter 4 for peripheral I.V. dressings and as specified in Chapter 5 for central I.V. dressings.
- The I.V. insertion site is assessed carefully during dressing changes and as per agency or hospital protocol for evidence of infection or phlebitis. This may be evidenced by erythema (i.e., redness), edema (i.e., swelling), streaking, purulent drainage, or finding a palpable venous cord at the insertion site. If any of these are present, they are graded using the *phlebitis scale*[6] noted on Table 6-1, the physician is notified, and the findings are documented in the patient's record.
- Vital signs are monitored as ordered for the patient, and any fever (e.g., temperature $\geq$ 100.4°F) in any patient or low temperature ($\leq$97.2°F) in a patient who is immunosuppressed is noted. The patient's physician is notified if any of these occur, and findings are documented in the patient's record.
- The white blood cell (WBC) count is scrutinized on the CBC when ordered. Infection is suspected in patients with elevated total WBCs (e.g., >11,000/mm^3) or decreased WBCs in patients who are immunosuppressed (e.g., <4000/mm^3). If a WBC differential is completed, a band count that comprises more than 10 percent of the sample suggests host invasion by bacterial microorganisms.
- The patient is taught principles and methods that can prevent infection, including that the I.V. dressing must be kept clean and dry, that the delivery system must stay intact and not be disconnected, and that any insertion-site pain or noteworthy changes in site appearance should be reported promptly.[19]

Table 6-1   The Phlebitis Scale[6]

Grade	Clinical Criteria
0	No symptoms
1	Erythema at access site with or without pain
2	Pain at access site with erythema and/or edema
3	Pain at access site with erythema and/or edema
	Streak formation
	Palpable venous cord
4	Pain at access site with erythema and/or edema
	Streak formation
	Palpable venous cord more than 1 inch in length
	Purulent drainage

RISK FOR INJURY

4 Patients who are prescribed I.V. therapy are at risk for externally induced injuries,[18] otherwise called *iatrogenic injuries*. Patients may be at risk for complications or adverse events that result from insertion of a venous access device, as a consequence of maintaining I.V. therapy, or when a venous access device is removed. Some of the most pertinent complications and adverse events include infection, infiltration, thrombosis, air embolism, pneumothorax, and hemothorax. Risk for infection has been discussed previously; therefore, this section will focus on the other specified complications. Expected outcomes include that patients will remain free from these injurious complications.[19] Nursing interventions revolve around ensuring vigilant surveillance and facilitating prompt collaborative action with the patient's physician if any of these complications occur. The nurse also plans interventions that are known to decrease the likelihood that the complications will occur.

Infiltration occurs when a vein that is used as an access site for an I.V. delivery system becomes fragile and is injured. I.V. solution then leaks into the surrounding tissue. This happens more commonly when access devices are placed in smaller, more fragile peripheral veins than when access devices are placed in central veins. The nurse monitors the I.V. site for infiltration:

- Whenever dressing changes are done

- Whenever the I.V. delivery system is changed

- Whenever the solution is not flowing properly or there is an apparent obstruction to flow

- Whenever the patient complains of pain or tenderness at the I.V. access site
- At intervals noted per agency or hospital protocol

The nurse should document the presence or absence of infiltration on the patient's record using the *infiltration scale*[6] that is displayed on Table 6-2. Whenever infiltration is suspected in a peripheral I.V. line, the line should be discontinued and begun again using a different vein. Warm compresses may be applied to the site of infiltration to alleviate discomfort and edema and to encourage the expeditious absorption of the infiltrate.[6] Suspected infiltration of a central I.V. line should be reported to the physician, and the data that support this suspicion should be documented in the patient's record.

Thrombosis occurs when a blood clot (i.e., a thrombus) forms on the venous access device.[6] Thrombi may form on any type of venous access device whether it uses a peripheral or central access site. Clinical manifestations of thrombosis tend to mimic those of phlebitis, and generally, the nursing interventions mirror the treatment for suspected infiltration of peripheral and central I.V. access devices. That is, whenever thrombus formation is suspected on a peripheral venous access device, the line is discontinued, and a new site is accessed using a fresh delivery setup and access device. The old access site is treated with a warm compress.[6] Suspected thrombus formation on a central access device should be reported promptly to the physician, and supporting evidence should be documented in the patient's record.

Thromboses might be prevented by periodically flushing access devices per agency or hospital protocol if patients are not receiving a continuous infusion. Flushes commonly used include saline (e.g., 0.9% normal saline [NS]) and heparinized flush solution (e.g., 100 units heparin/mL). Thrombi can become dislodged and become emboli, which may cause target-organ damage. Peripheral thrombi rarely are associated with significant target-organ damage. However, thrombi that form from central venous access sites can dislodge and become emboli that then rapidly travel from the central venous vasculature to the right side of the heart and into the pulmonary vasculature, causing pulmonary ischemia, pulmonary infarction, and eventually, pulmonary necrosis. This may be manifested by dyspnea, confusion, hemoptysis, and respiratory failure.

Air emboli may form in the venous vasculature whenever air inappropriately infuses into the vein via the I.V. delivery system. This may occur if there are air bubbles in the solution that are not flushed out before infusion into the patient. A few small air bubbles rarely cause any significant complications when they infuse into a peripheral vein because vascular flow breaks up the air bubble before it reaches the central vasculature. If air bubbles infuse into a central I.V. line, however, this can cause serious injury because a pulmonary embolus may form, leading to a

Table 6-2   The Infiltration Scale[6]

Grade	Clinical Criteria
0	No symptoms
1	Skin blanched
	Edema less than 1 inch in any direction
	Skin cool to touch
	With or without pain
2	Skin blanched
	Edema from 1–6 inches in any direction
	Skin cool to touch
	With or without pain
3	Skin blanched, translucent
	Gross edema more than 6 inches in any direction
	Skin cool to touch
	Mild to moderate pain
	Possible numbness
4	Skin blanched, translucent
	Skin tight, leaking
	Skin discolored, bruised, swollen
	Gross edema more than 6 inches in any direction
	Deep pitting tissue edema
	Circulatory impairment
	Moderate to severe pain
	Infiltration of any amount of blood product, irritant, or vesicant

pulmonary infarction and pulmonary necrosis. Whenever central I.V. lines are initiated, disconnected, or discontinued, normal changes in intrathoracic pressure that occur during the respiratory cycle can result in air being drawn into the access site. This is another key cause of air embolus formation. This may be prevented by coaching the patient to perform the Valsalva maneuver whenever a central I.V. line setup is initiated, changed, or discontinued.[6]

Pneumothorax and hemothorax are serious complications that can occur during insertion of a central venous access device.[6] Pneumothorax is caused when the introducer used to gain central venous access inadvertently punctures the pleural space, resulting in air being pulled into that space and causing partial or total collapse of the lung on the side of the injury. Hemothorax may occur if a vessel is punctured during this process, causing blood to fill the pleural space, and the lung then collapses. Both pneumothorax and hemothorax may be manifested by dyspnea, respiratory distress, hypoxemia, and eventual cardiopulmonary collapse if emergent decisive action is not taken, including the insertion of a chest tube.

RISK FOR DISUSE SYNDROME

4 Patients with peripheral I.V. access sites that are located close to joints may have restricted mobility and may need to use arm boards to ensure that the venous access device remains stable and intact. When this occurs, these patients may be at risk for disuse syndrome, which can be manifested by weakness of the muscles around that joint and possible muscle atrophy.[18] Therefore, the expected outcome for patients who must use arm boards or other types of ancillary devices that limit mobility because of the location of their venous access devices is that muscle weakness and atrophy will not occur.[19] An obvious nursing intervention that can prevent disuse syndrome is to select a venous access site that is not located near a joint.[6] If it is necessary to place a venous access device close to a joint, then the nurse can intervene to prevent disuse syndrome by removing the arm board or immobilizing device periodically to assess musculoskeletal integrity and by having the patient periodically contract and relax the at-risk muscles without moving the joint.

ANXIETY

4 Anxiety is experienced commonly by patients who are prescribed I.V. therapy, particularly during initiation of I.V. access. Many patients will tell the nurse that they are anxious about having venipuncture performed and a venous access device inserted. Evidence that also can support the nursing diagnosis of anxiety includes the following patient manifestations:

Behavioral manifestations

- Scanning and vigilance
- Poor eye contact
- Restlessness
- Fidgeting

Affective manifestations

- Irritability
- Increased wariness
- Worried, apprehensive

Physiological manifestations

- Voice quivering
- Trembling, shakiness
- Increased perspiration
- Facial tension
- Faintness[18]

The patient's anxiety may be related to stress or to perceived threats to the patient's health status and interactive patterns.[18] An appropriate expected outcome is that the patient copes appropriately with I.V. initiation and maintenance therapy.[19] Nursing interventions that may help the patient cope appropriately include discussing the nature of the procedure in advance with the patient and answering any questions the patient may have, thus offering anticipatory guidance. Relaxation and distraction also may be appropriate nursing interventions while venipuncture is being performed and the venous access device is inserted.[19]

DEFICIENT KNOWLEDGE

4   Many patients prescribed I.V. therapy have never had an I.V. line placed previously and do not understand the rationale for its placement, do not know methods they may take to ensure its safe maintenance, and do not understand how I.V. therapy may benefit them. They may tell the nurse that they do not understand why they need an I.V. line placed or express fear or bewilderment over their role in ensuring that the I.V. administration setup is maintained as prescribed. Expected outcomes for these patients are that they verbalize appropriate knowledge of both the I.V. initiation procedure and their role in ensuring maintenance of the therapeutic I.V. regimen.[19]

Appropriate nursing interventions for patients who have I.V. access devices placed would include explaining to the patient the rationale for the therapy and how the I.V. therapy will help improve their overall health status and teaching them methods they may use to prevent complications from occurring.[19]

Summary

The professional nurse uses the nursing process when rendering care to a patient prescribed I.V. therapy. Actual and potential nursing diagnoses form a framework for planning care for these patients. Identifying the actual and potential nursing diagnoses that are particularly salient for patients who receive I.V. therapy helps nurses to focus their plans of care appropriately.

Quiz

1. Which of the following is *not* a common NANDA nursing diagnosis for a patient prescribed I.V. therapy?

   (a) Deficient fluid volume

   (b) Risk for disuse syndrome

   (c) Anxiety

   (d) Decreased cardiac output

2. Patients at risk for deficient fluid volume would include *all but which* of the following?

   (a) Patients unable to self-hydrate

   (b) Patients with dry mucus membranes

   (c) Patients prescribed diuretic agents

   (d) Patients scheduled for major surgery

3. Clinical manifestations that might suggest phlebitis at the venous access site include which of the following?

   (a) Blanched skin

   (b) Numbness

   (c) Skin cool to touch

   (d) Purulent drainage

4. Which of the following complications is *least likely* to occur when a central venous access device is used rather than a peripheral venous access device?

   (a) Infiltration

   (b) Air embolism

   (c) Pneumothorax

   (d) Hemothorax

5. Which of the following statements about disuse syndrome is true?

   (a) Disuse syndrome may be prevented by choosing a peripheral access site that is not in close proximity to a joint.

   (b) Disuse syndrome always results in atrophy of muscles.

   (c) Disuse syndrome may be prevented by periodically flushing venous access devices with heparin flush solution (e.g., 100 units heparin/mL).

   (d) Disuse syndrome may be prevented by encouraging the patient to flex and extend the immobilized joint periodically.

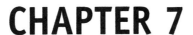

CHAPTER 7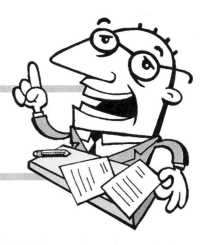

Crystalloid Solutions

Learning Objectives

After completing this chapter, the learner will

1. Discuss the characteristics of various types of crystalloid solutions.

2. Differentiate isotonic, hypotonic, and hypertonic crystalloid solutions from each other.

3. Compare and contrast the initial response and the therapeutic response that occur when crystalloids are infused intravenously.

4. Discuss indications for use of common crystalloid solutions.

5. Identify adverse events that may occur when common crystalloid solutions are infused intravenously.

Key Terms

Crystalloids
Initial response
Therapeutic response

Crystalloids Defined

1 **Crystalloids** are types of intravenous (I.V.) solutions that contain solutes dissolved in water.[20] These solutes may include dextrose, electrolytes, or a combination of both. Crystalloids are described in terms of their tonicity as compared with plasma. They are also classified according to their composition as sodium solutions, dextrose solutions, or mixed electrolyte solutions. Because crystalloids are not particularly viscous, they can be administered rapidly through both peripheral and central I.V. lines.[21] Crystalloids are administered most commonly either to correct or to prevent fluid and electrolyte disturbances. Once administered into the vasculature, crystalloids tend to distribute their concentration rapidly in a manner that mirrors the physiologic distribution of fluids into the intracellular and extracellular fluid compartments depending on the tonicity of the solution.[21]

SPEED BUMP

The most common indication for prescribing intravenous (I.V.) infusions of crystalloids is to correct or prevent _____ disturbances.

Tonicity of Solutions

The term *tonicity* was defined in Chapter 2 as a measure of osmotically active particles in a given solution for a unit of mass. Tonicity refers to the ability of a given solution to generate osmotic pressure. **2** Crystalloids that have a tonicity that is similar to that of plasma are considered isotonic because they generate little osmotic pressure. Simplistically, this means that isotonic fluids have little appreciable effect on cells that come into contact with them. On the other hand, solutions that are hypotonic and hypertonic do generate osmotic pressure-gradient changes between the extracellular and intracellular environments. Cells that come into contact with hypotonic solutions tend to swell, whereas cells that come into contact

Table 7-1   Tonicity and Electrolyte and Dextrose Composition of Commonly
Prescribed Crystalloids

Isotonic Solutions	mOsm/L	Na+ (mEq/L)	K+ (mEq/L)	Cl- (mEq/L)	Ca2+ (mEq/L)	Lactate (mEq/L)	Dextrose (gm/dL)
Saline (0.9% NS)	308	154		154			
5% dextrose in water (D_5W)	280						5
Ringer's	310	147		155	4		
Lactated Ringer's (LR)	275	130	4	109	3	28	
Hypotonic Solutions	**mOsm/L**	**Na+ (mEq/L)**	**K+ (mEq/L)**	**Cl- (mEq/L)**	**Ca2+ (mEq/L)**	**Lactate (mEq/L)**	**Dextrose (g/dL)**
Half-normal saline (0.45% NS)	155	77		77			
Hypertonic Solutions	**mOsm/L**	**Na+ (mEq/L)**	**K+ (mEq/L)**	**Cl- (mEq/L)**	**Ca2+ (mEq/L)**	**Lactate (mEq/L)**	**Dextrose (g/dL)**
3% Sodium chloride (3% NS)	1030	513		513			
10% Dextrose in water ($D_{10}W$)	505						10
5% Dextrose–half-normal saline ($D_5$0.45% NS)	406	77		77			5
5% Dextrose–normal saline ($D_5$0.9% NS)	560	154		154			5
5% Dextrose–lactated Ringer's (D_5LR)	527	130	4	109	3	28	5

with hypertonic solutions tend to shrink.[22] Table 7-1 lists the osmolalities of commonly prescribed isotonic, hypotonic, and hypertonic crystalloid solutions and their respective electrolyte and dextrose contents.

ISOTONIC SOLUTIONS

Isotonic solutions have a tonicity that is similar to that of plasma. The osmolality of plasma is approximately 285 mOsm/L, and it has an approximate electrolyte content of 310 mEq/L. Crystalloids are considered isotonic if their osmolality ranges between 275 and 310 mOsm/L. Examples of these include saline (i.e., 0.9% normal saline [NS]), lactated Ringer's (LR) solution, and 5% dextrose in water (D_5W).[22]

HYPOTONIC SOLUTIONS

Hypotonic solutions have a tonicity that is less than that of plasma with an osmolality that is less than 275 mOsm/L and an electrolyte content that is less than 250 mEq/L. As noted in Chapter 2, when cells have a greater osmolality than the solutions that surround them, osmotic pressure is generated, and fluid moves across the cell membranes and into the cells, causing cellular swelling. Examples of commonly prescribed hypotonic solutions include free water and half-normal saline (i.e., 0.45% NS).

HYPERTONIC SOLUTIONS

Hypertonic solutions have a tonicity that is greater than that of plasma with an osmolality greater than 310 mOsm/L and an electrolyte content that exceeds 375 mEq/L. Cells bathed in a milieu of a hypertonic solution behave the opposite of those in contact with a hypotonic solution. That is, osmotic pressure is indeed generated when cells come into contact with a solution that has a greater osmolality than the osmolality of their intracellular fluid. However, in these cases, intracellular fluid tends to shift by osmosis across the cell membrane into the extracellular environment, causing cellular shrinking. An example of a commonly prescribed hypertonic solution is 5% dextrose in saline (i.e., $D_5 0.9\%$ NS).[12,22]

Physiologic Responses to Crystalloid Infusions

Crystalloids come into immediate contact with blood cells when they are infused intravenously. They also come into contact with the cells that line the vascular endothelium, which are the cells that line the inner layer of the vasculature and that interface directly with blood. **3** The blood cells and endothelial cells tend to respond in some way to their contact with the crystalloid solution. This is referred to as the **initial response**.[20] The nature of how the crystalloid solution eventually disperses itself into the body's fluid compartments is referred to as the **therapeutic response**.[20]

INITIAL RESPONSE

The nature of the initial response depends mostly on the tonicity of the crystalloid that is infused intravenously. As noted previously, hypotonic solutions cause cells that come in contact with them to swell. Therefore, blood cells and vascular endothelial cells that come in contact with hypotonic solutions swell. Half-normal saline (i.e., 0.45% NS) is a hypotonic solution that can cause this type of initial response. Conversely, blood cells and vascular endothelial cells that come into contact with hypertonic solutions may shrink. Hypertonic solutions that may cause this type of initial response may include 3% sodium chloride (3% NaCl), 10% dextrose in water (D_{10}W), 5% dextrose in half-normal saline ($D_5 0.45\%$ NS), 5% dextrose in normal saline ($D_5 0.9\%$ NS), and 5% dextrose in lactated Ringers solution (D₅LR). In either case, cell function is hampered, and cell lysis and death may occur if the solution is either highly hypotonic or hypertonic.[20]

A clear advantage to using isotonic solutions is that the integrity of blood cells and endothelial cells is not compromised. However, there are therapeutic indications for prescribing hypotonic and hypertonic solutions. For instance, in cases of hypernatremia, the cells are at risk of shrinking, and cellular lysis may occur. Administering a solution such as D₅W actually may have the therapeutic effect of causing cellular rehydration. Conversely, in cases of hyponatremia, the cells tend to swell and become damaged. Administering a hypertonic solution such as 3% NS can have the favorable effect of diminishing cellular swelling and correcting the hyponatremia.[20]

Speed Bump

The nature of the initial response depends mostly on the _____ of the fluid that is infused intravenously.

THERAPEUTIC RESPONSE

Crystalloids tend to be dextrose- or electrolyte-based solutions or a combination of both. The solutions that are electrolyte-based are either primarily sodium-based (e.g., 0.9% NS or saline) or contain multiple electrolytes (e.g., LR). Saline and LR are isotonic solutions. Therefore, their therapeutic response mirrors the physiologic distribution of fluids in the extracellular fluid, and 75 percent of the fluid infused rapidly disperses into the interstitial space, whereas 25 percent of the fluid infused remains within the intravascular space. Therefore, for each liter of saline or LR that is infused, 750 mL disperses into the interstitial space and 250 mL remains within the vascular compartment.

Although D₅W is considered an isotonic solution, it behaves much differently at the physiologic level during the therapeutic response than either saline or LR. The dextrose in the solution becomes consumed by the cells, and eventually, only free water remains. Water is hypotonic compared with intracellular fluid, and the cells respond by swelling. The actual dispersion of the water into fluid compartments is predictable because, once again, it mimics distribution of fluids into the intracellular and extracellular fluid compartments at the physiologic level. Approximately two-thirds of the water will disperse intracellularly, whereas the remaining one-third of the water will stay within the extracellular fluid (ECF) compartment. Thus, for each liter of D₅W infused, 667 mL will disperse into the intracellular fluid (ICF) compartment and 333 mL will disperse into the ECF compartment. Of the 333 mL of water dispersed into the ECF, approximately 75 percent will disperse to the interstitium (i.e., 250 mL), whereas only 25 percent will remain within the intravascular space (i.e., 83 mL).[20]

Many crystalloid solutions contain a combination of dextrose and electrolytes. A commonly prescribed combination solution is $D_5 0.45\%$ NS. This solution is considered hypertonic, with an approximate osmolality of 406 mOsm/L. However, once the cells consume the dextrose in this solution, the balance of solution remaining is half saline and half free water, which is slightly hypotonic. Thus it can be predicted that for each liter of $D_5 0.45\%$ NS infused, half the solution eventually will disperse in the manner of free water, and half eventually will disperse in the manner of saline into the respective fluid compartments. Eventually, 333 mL of fluid will disperse into the ICF compartment, 500 mL of fluid will disperse into the interstitium, and 167 mL of fluid will remain in the vascular space.[20]

Another commonly prescribed hypertonic solution that contains a mix of both dextrose and electrolytes is $D_5 0.9\%$ NS. This crystalloid solution has an osmolality of 560 mOsm/L. Once again, the dextrose in the solution is consumed soon after it is infused by the host's cells; when this occurs, the solution that remains is saline (0.9% NS), which is isotonic. Therefore, for each liter of $D_5 0.9\%$ NS infused, 750 mL eventually will disperse to the interstitial space, and 250 mL will remain in the vascular space. $D_5 LR$, another hypertonic solution with an osmolality of 527 mOsm/L, behaves in exactly the same manner. That is, once the dextrose in solution is consumed, the remaining LR behaves as an isotonic solution and distributes 75 percent of the infused solution into the interstitium, with distribution of the remaining 25 percent within the vascular compartment.

Composition of Solutions

Crystalloid solutions are classified based on their tonicity and their composite solutes. Most crystalloids are sodium-based solutions, dextrose-based solutions, mixed-electrolyte solutions, or a combination of any of these. Combination solutions tend to contain both dextrose and sodium or both dextrose and mixed electrolytes. Most combination solutions tend to be hypertonic and behave as described earlier in terms of therapeutic response.

SODIUM SOLUTIONS

Sodium-based crystalloids may be isotonic (e.g., saline or 0.9% NS), hypotonic (e.g., half-normal saline or 0.45% NS), or hypertonic (e.g., 3% NS). Saline is sometimes referred to as *normal saline* because its osmolality closely mirrors that of plasma. **4** It is the crystalloid that has the least risk of causing hemolysis of red blood cells and therefore is the flush solution of choice when blood transfusions are given. It is also indicated to replenish or support circulatory volume during states of shock or in acute conditions that may result in shock states, including severe dehydration, diabetic ketoacidosis, burns, and adrenal insufficiency.[23] **5** Complications associated with overzealous infusion of saline may include fluid overload, hypokalemia and dilution of other key electrolytes, and hyperchloremic acidosis.[13,22]

4 Indications for prescribing I.V. infusions of half-normal saline (i.e., 0.45% NS) generally revolve around conditions that result in cellular dehydration. Examples of conditions that might result in cellular dehydration include overzealous use of diuretic agents, excessive vomiting, and hyperglycemic hyperosmolar nonketotic coma.[23] **5** Complications that may arise from infusion of half-normal saline include hyponatremia and cellular overhydration and swelling.[22]

4 Hypertonic sodium chloride I.V. solutions (e.g., 3% NS) are prescribed most commonly to treat severe hyponatremia that may result from renal failure, excessive diaphoresis, or excessive intake of free water. **5** Patients who receive infusions of hypertonic sodium chloride are at heightened risk of suffering circulatory overload. This solution also irritates peripheral veins and should be administered slowly to prevent both venous irritation and circulatory overload.[24]

DEXTROSE SOLUTIONS

Dextrose-based crystalloids tend to be composed of varying amounts of dextrose in free water. The most commonly prescribed dextrose-based solution is 5% dextrose in water (D_5W). As discussed previously, D_5W is an isotonic solution with an osmolality of 280 mOsm/L. However, once the dextrose dissolved in this solution is metabolized by the body cells, the free water that remains from the original solution behaves like a hypotonic solution. **4** Indications for I.V. infusion of this solution therefore include hyperosmolar states and hypernatremia.[20] The dextrose in this solution provides minimal caloric content (170 kcal/L) that may help to avert ketosis in patients who are NPO. The dextrose also serves to facilitate the transport of potassium from the extracellular into the intracellular environment, thereby promoting electrolyte balance in both the ICF and ECF compartments.[23]

There are other dextrose-based solutions of variable concentration dissolved in free water, including, for instance, 10% dextrose in water ($D_{10}W$) and 50% dextrose in water ($D_{50}W$). These solutions tend to behave as highly hypertonic solutions when first infused and generally are administered for the treatment of hypoglycemia. **5** Because dextrose-based solutions tend to be quite acidic, with pH values that range from 3.4 to 4.0, they can irritate peripheral veins when they are infused. Complications that may occur as a result of I.V. infusion of dextrose-based infusions include hyperglycemia, hyponatremia, and water intoxication. In addition, highly concentrated dextrose solutions may cause an osmotic diuresis with resulting dehydration.[22,23]

MIXED-ELECTROLYTE SOLUTIONS

Ringer's and lactated Ringer's solutions are commonly prescribed mixed-electrolyte solutions. Both are isotonic solutions that may be prescribed when fluid is depleted within the vascular compartment, as may occur in shock states or conditions that result in shock. Lactated Ringer's (LR) solution is sometimes also called *Hartmann's solution*. Both LR and Ringer's solutions contain concentrations of multiple electrolytes that are similar to the composition of plasma. **4** However, LR tends to be prescribed more frequently than Ringer's because it also contains lactate. Lactate metabolizes into bicarbonate, which buffers the acidity of the solution and may partially correct the metabolic acidosis that ensues in states of shock. Because of this, LR is preferred by some clinicians as the crystalloid of choice for treating shock states over not only Ringer's but also saline, which can cause a hyperchloremic acidosis. However, LR is contraindicated in patients with liver disease because lactate is metabolized in the liver. **5** Complications that may result from I.V. LR therapy include hypoglycemia, hypernatremia, and fluid overload, as well as, in rare cases, metabolic alkalosis.[22,24]

Summary

Crystalloids are indicated as fluids of choice to treat or prevent fluid and electrolyte deficits. Crystalloid solutions are classified in terms of their tonicity and the composition of their solutes, which may include electrolytes and/or dextrose. The eventual dispersion of fluids into the intracellular, interstitial, and intravascular compartments occurs during the therapeutic response and can be quantified and predicted.

Quiz

1. Crystalloids that have a tonicity that closely mirrors the tonicity of plasma are referred to as

   (a) hypotonic solutions.

   (b) isotonic solutions.

   (c) hypertonic solutions.

   (d) eutonic solutions.

2. Which of the following is the crystalloid of choice for use as a flush solution during blood transfusions?

   (a) Saline (0.9% NS)

   (b) D_5W

   (c) LR

   (d) Ringer's

3. Five percent dextrose in water (D_5W) is classified as

   (a) a hypotonic solution.

   (b) an isotonic solution.

   (c) a hypertonic solution.

   (d) a mixed-electrolyte solution.

4. During the therapeutic response that occurs after D_5W is infused, the fluid infused behaves as if it were which type of solution?

   (a) A hypotonic solution

   (b) An isotonic solution

   (c) A hypertonic solution

   (d) A mixed-electrolyte solution

5. A patient who receives a 500-mL infusion of LR likely will have a net gain of how many milliliters of fluid into the vascular compartment during the therapeutic response?

   (a) 375 mL

   (b) 250 mL

   (c) 125 mL

   (d) None

6. A patient who receives a 500-mL infusion of LR will have a net gain of how many milliliters of fluid into the interstitium during the therapeutic response?

   (a) 375 mL

   (b) 250 mL

   (c) 125 mL

   (d) None

7. A patient who receives a 500-mL infusion of LR will have a net gain of how many milliliters of fluid into the intracellular compartment during the therapeutic response?

   (a) 375 mL

   (b) 250 mL

   (c) 125 mL

   (d) None

8. A patient receives a 3000-mL infusion of $D_5 0.45\%$ NS over 24 hours. This type of solution is considered

   (a) isotonic.

   (b) hypotonic.

   (c) hypertonic.

   (d) eutonic.

9. A patient receives a 3000-mL infusion of $D_5 0.45\%$ NS over 24 hours. Which of the following best describes what happens during the initial response to this therapy?

   (a) The blood cells and vascular endothelial cells are not affected by coming in contact with the solution.

   (b) The blood cells and vascular endothelial cells swell when they come into contact with the solution.

   (c) The blood cells and vascular endothelial cells shrink when they come into contact with the solution.

   (d) The blood cells and vascular endothelial cells consume the 0.45% NS solution on contact.

10. A patient receives 3000 mL of $D_5 0.45\%$ NS in 24 hours. How much of this solution remains in the intravascular space during the therapeutic response?

   (a) 167 mL

   (b) 500 mL

   (c) 501 mL

   (d) 999 mL

11. A patient receives 3000 mL of $D_5 0.45\%$ NS in 24 hours. How much of this solution disperses to the intracellular space during the therapeutic response?

   (a) 167 mL

   (b) 500 mL

   (c) 501 mL

   (d) 999 mL

12. A patient receives a bolus of 500 mL of LR over 30 minutes. Which of the following best describes the initial response to this infusion?

   (a) The blood cells and vascular endothelial cells are not affected by coming in contact with the solution.

   (b) The blood cells and vascular endothelial cells swell when they come into contact with the solution.

   (c) The blood cells and vascular endothelial cells shrink when they come into contact with the solution.

   (d) The blood cells and vascular endothelial cells consume the lactate in the solution on contact.

13. A patient receives a bolus of 500 mL of LR over 30 minutes. Which of the following best describes the therapeutic response to this infusion?

   (a) 0 mL of solution disperses into the intracellular space, 375 mL of solution disperses to the interstitium, and 125 mL of solution remain in the intravascular space.

   (b) 333 mL of solution disperses into the intracellular space, 167 mL of solution disperses to the interstitium, and 0 mL of solution remains in the intravascular space.

   (c) 333 mL of solution disperses into the intracellular space, 125 mL of solution disperses to the interstitium, and 42 mL of solution remains in the intravascular space.

   (d) 500 mL of solution remains in the intravascular space.

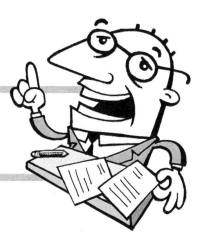

CHAPTER 8

Colloid Solutions

Learning Objectives

After completing this chapter, the learner will

1. Compare and contrast the characteristics of colloid solutions with crystalloid solutions.

2. Differentiate nonsynthetic and synthetic colloid solutions.

3. Discuss indications for use of common colloid solutions.

4. Identify adverse effects that may occur from utilizing common colloid solutions.

 Key Terms

Colloids	Hespan
Albumin	Dextran
Plasma protein fraction (PPF)	

Colloids Defined

Colloids are types of intravenous (I.V.) solutions that contain macromolecules and electrolytes. **1** Colloid solutions have a significantly higher molecular weight than crystalloid solutions. The macromolecules contained in colloid solutions characteristically do not pass readily through membranes, including capillary membranes and cellular membranes, in their normal, healthy state. Therefore, colloids behave differently at a physiologic level from crystalloids because when colloids are infused intravenously, they generate colloidal osmotic pressure (COP).[25]

Because colloids maintain and also can generate or enhance COP, colloid solutions tend to stay within the intravascular compartment rather than cause fluid shifts into the interstitium or the intracellular fluid (ICF) compartment. As a general rule of thumb, each milliliter of colloids infused into the intravascular space remains within the intravascular space. Some colloids have the added effect of drawing additional fluid from the interstitium into the intravascular space. When colloids are infused and supplemented with isotonic crystalloids such as lactated Ringer's (LR) or normal saline (0.9% NS), the net effect is that additional fluid remains within the vasculature. For these reasons, colloids are referred to frequently as *volume expanders* or *plasma expanders*.

SPEED BUMP

Colloid solutions can be distinguished from crystalloid solutions because colloid solutions may generate _____ when they are infused into the vasculature.

Types of Colloids

2 Colloids can be classified as either nonsynthetic or synthetic. Nonsynthetic colloids are derived from human blood components. Synthetic colloids are biomedically manufactured from nonhuman sources.

NONSYNTHETIC COLLOIDS

Nonsynthetic colloids tend to be derived from human plasma. The most commonly used nonsynthetic colloids are composed primarily of albumin, which is the major plasma protein. These include albumin 5% (i.e., Plasbumin-5) and albumin 25% (i.e., Plasbumin-25) and plasma protein fraction (i.e., Plasmanate).

SYNTHETIC COLLOIDS

Synthetic colloids are derived from gelatins, dextrans, and starches. Examples of gelatin colloids include urea-bridged gelatin and modified-fluid gelatin. Starches include hetastarch (i.e., Hespan) and pentastarch (i.e., Pentaspan). Dextrans include such colloid solutions as Dextran-40 and Dextran-70. Synthetic colloids generally tend to carry more risks of causing adverse reactions than do nonsynthetic colloids.[25] Colloids are more expensive than crystalloids, and albumin is the most expensive colloid.

Indications for the Use of Colloids

3   Colloids are very effective at either replacing or expanding vascular volume in patients who are hypovolemic. They tend to be infused in tandem with isotonic crystalloids such as normal saline and lactated Ringer's solution. When infused simultaneously, colloids and isotonic crystalloids are quite effective at mitigating clinical manifestations of hypovolemia, including hypovolemic shock. Table 8-1 lists the causes of hypovolemic shock and early signs and symptoms of hypovolemic shock.

Table 8-1   Hypovolemic Shock

Cause	Clinical Manifestations
Hemorrhage (i.e., hemorrhagic shock)	Neurologic
Burns (i.e., burn shock)	Anxiety
Dehydration from	Restlessness or agitation
Excessive vomiting	Disorientation
Excessive diarrhea	Cardiovascular
Excessive sweating	Tachycardia
Polyuria (e.g., diabetes insipidus,	Narrowed pulse pressure
diabetic ketoacidosis [DKA],	Orthostasis
hyperosmolar hyperglycemic	Hypotension
nonketotic coma [HHNK],	Prolonged capillary refill
overzealous use of diuretics)	Pulmonary
	Tachypnea
	Air hunger
	Renal
	Oliguria
	Dermatologic
	Cool, clammy skin
	Mottling

Evidence from research studies do not clearly demonstrate improved outcomes in patients fluid-resuscitated with colloids and crystalloids over those fluid-resuscitated without colloids.[25] However, patients who exhibit manifestations of hypovolemic shock as a consequence of hemodialysis do tend to demonstrate improved outcomes with infusions of colloids,[25] and colloids therefore are indicated in this subset of patients with hypovolemia.

Colloids also may be infused prophylactically to prevent shock or loss of intravascular volume or to encourage stabilization of vascular volume. For instance, patients with burn shock tend to exhibit capillary membrane instability during the first 24 hours after the burn. As a result of this, much of the plasma proteins seep into the interstitium and draw plasma fluid into the interstitium with them by osmosis. The capillary membranes begin to stabilize 24 hours after the burn. Intravenous infusions of albumin help to draw fluid back into the vascular compartment from the interstitium.

Because colloids are effective at expanding vascular volume, the nurse must monitor patients who receive I.V. colloids closely for clinical manifestations of circulatory overload and pulmonary edema,[20] particularly elderly patients and patients with a known history of heart failure. These signs and symptoms are summarized in Table 8-2.

Table 8-2 Clinical Manifestations of Circulatory Overload

System	Common Sign	Common Symptom
Neurologic	Restlessness	Disorientation
	Agitation	Anxiety
Cardiovascular	S_3	
	S_4	
	New murmur or increased grade (i.e., intensity) of previous murmur	
	Tachycardia	
	Orthostasis	
	Hypotension	
	Prolonged capillary refill	
Pulmonary	Bibasilar rales	Orthopnea
	Pink, frothy sputum	Air hunger
	Hypoxemia	Paroxysmal nocturnal dyspnea (PND)
Renal	Oliguria	
Dermatologic	Cold, clammy skin	
	Mottling	

SPEED BUMP

SPEED BUMP

Colloids are indicated mainly to treat or prevent _____.

Albumin

Albumin (i.e., Plasbumin) is derived from pooled human plasma. It is simply a sterile solution of human albumin suspended in an aqueous diluent.[26] Each vial of albumin contains approximately 145 mEq/L of the electrolyte sodium. Albumin is the major plasma protein and, as such, is the molecule that is primarily responsible for maintaining colloidal osmotic pressure (COP).

Albumin is also a transport molecule. This means that albumin can bind to many other molecules, including bilirubin, metals, enzymes, drugs, and electrolytes, and transport or inactivate them.[11] For instance, because hydrogen ion binds readily with albumin, albumin can act as a buffer in solution. Likewise, patients who are hypoalbuminemic are at heightened risk for acidosis because there is proportionately less albumin to bind with hydrogen ion.

Two concentrations of albumin are available commercially for I.V. infusions. The first is albumin 5% (i.e., Plasbumin-5). This colloid is osmotically similar to plasma and is isotonic with an approximate osmolality of 290 mOsm/L.[25] As albumin 5% is osmotically similar to plasma, 1 mL of fluid will be retained in the vascular compartment for each milliliter of albumin 5% infused intravenously.

The second concentration of albumin that is available commercially for I.V. infusion is albumin 25% (i.e., Plasbumin-25). This colloidal solution is hyperosmotic and hypertonic and will draw additional fluid from the interstitium into the vascular compartment. It can generate COP of approximately 70 to 100 mm Hg. The COP generated by albumin 25% can result in a net gain of up to 4 mL of vascular volume for each milliliter of albumin 25% infused.[27]

Vials that contain both albumin 5% and albumin 25% should be stored at room temperature. Each vial should be examined prior to use to ensure that it is not cracked and that there is no visible turbidity of the solution. Infusions should be completed within 4 hours after the vial is accessed; any residual solution should be discarded. Table 8-3 lists the volume and albumin concentration contained in commercially available vials of both albumin 5% and albumin 25%.

INDICATIONS

3 Albumin 5% may be indicated for use in patients who are hypovolemic for a variety of reasons, including hemorrhage, burns, and dehydration. Albumin 25% may be indicated for use in these same patients if their COP is low, which may

Table 8-3 Commercially Available Vials of Albumin

Concentration	Volume	Albumin Composition
Albumin 5%	50 mL	2.5 g
	250 mL	12.5 g
	500 mL	25.0 g
Albumin 25%	20 mL	5.0 g
	50 mL	12.5 g
	100 mL	25.0 g

occur in severe states of shock. In these instances, albumin 25% should be accompanied by crystalloids and perhaps diuretics to encourage vascular volume expansion and adequate renal glomerular filtration.[22]

Albumin infusions typically are withheld from patients with severe burns until at least 24 hours after the burn, when it is believed that the capillary membrane has stabilized physiologically and the albumin will not pool in the interstitium. The use of albumin in patients who have lost a lot of blood should not precede attempts at hemodynamic stabilization with crystalloids and blood component products if they are available. Albumin infusions can be particularly therapeutic in patients with liver failure that is accompanied by ascites and hyperbilirubinemia. In these patients, albumin has the net effect of pulling fluid from the interstitium, thereby reducing ascites. In addition, bilirubin binds to albumin, thereby diminishing serum free bilirubin levels.[26,27] Similarly, I.V. administration of albumin may reduce the interstitial edema that can occur with peritonitis and pancreatitis.[26,27]

ADVERSE EFFECTS

4 Because albumin is obtained from pooled human plasma, it can cause infections and allergic reactions. Viral infections may be transmitted from plasma, particularly hepatitis C. The risk of transmission of viruses via albumin infusions is less now than a few years ago because of improved donor selection methods and because the donated plasma is heat-treated during the separation process.[26,27]

In addition to viral infection, albumin I.V. infusions infrequently cause allergic or anaphylactic reactions. Common manifestations of an allergic reaction include flushing, urticaria, and chills.[26,27] If the patient is still receiving the infusion when an allergic reaction is suspected, the infusion should be discontinued immediately.

Likewise, albumin infusions are contraindicated in patients with a known hypersensitivity to albumin.

Albumin is also contraindicated in patients with nephrotic syndrome, which is characterized by renal glomerular instability and excretion of albumin in the urine.[26,27] Patients who receive angiotensin-converting enzyme (ACE) inhibitors concurrent with I.V. infusions of albumin are prone to experience flushing and hypotension. Therefore, whenever possible, ACE inhibitors should be withheld for 24 hours prior to the I.V. infusion of albumin. Although albumin had been used decades ago as therapy for patients who were malnourished, the advent of improved parenteral nutrition solutions and enteral nutrients has supplanted this indication for albumin (see Chapter 10 for a more complete discussion of parenteral nutrition therapy).

Plasma Protein Fraction

Plasma protein fraction 5% (i.e., Plasmanate) is derived from pooled human plasma and refined by electrophoresis. It is physiologically similar in composition and behavior to albumin. **Plasma protein fraction (PPF)** is composed of approximately 88 percent albumin, 12 percent alpha and beta globulins, and less than 1 percent gamma globulin. It is osmotically equivalent to human plasma and is isotonic. It contains approximately 145 mEq/L sodium, 0.25 mEq/L potassium, and 100 mEq/L chloride.[26] Table 8-4 lists the sizes of commercially available vials of PPF and their respective composition of proteins.

PPF should be stored at room temperature. Prior to use, the vial should be examined and if the vial is cracked or the solution appears turbid, it should not be used. In general, the infusion should be completed within 4 hours after the rubber stopper of the vial has been punctured. Unused solution should be discarded. Infusion rates should not exceed 10 mL/minute (i.e., 600 mL/h) or hypotension may occur.

Table 8-4   Commercially Available Vials of Plasma Protein Fraction

Plasma Protein Fraction	Volume	Protein Composition
	50 mL	2.5 g
	250 mL	12.5 g
	500 mL	25.0 g

INDICATIONS

3 PPF is indicated for the treatment of severe burns and, in some cases, hemorrhagic shock. PPF treatment for burns does not begin until at least 24 hours after the burn, when the capillary membranes have stabilized. Treatment of hemorrhagic shock with any colloid, including PPF, is controversial and should not supplant the use of crystalloids or blood component products.

ADVERSE EFFECTS

4 Because PPF is made from human plasma, it may contain organisms that can cause infectious diseases, such as viruses. Although screening of donors and testing of donated blood have diminished the risk of transmission of viruses through administration of PPF over the past several years, there is still a risk of transmission of some viruses, particularly hepatitis C.[26]

PPF also can cause allergic or anaphylactic reactions. Side effects of administration of PPF are frequent and may include flushing, back pain, nausea, headache, urticaria, chills, and fever. Sometimes these manifestations indicate a hypersensitivity reaction, and sometimes they are idiopathic (i.e., the cause is unknown). PPF is contraindicated for use in patients on cardiopulmonary bypass because it can cause hypotension in this population.[22]

Hespan

Hetastarches are large carbohydrate molecules. The most common hetastarch used as an I.V. colloidal solution is 6% hetastarch in 0.9% sodium chloride solution, otherwise known as **Hespan** or *hydroxyethyl starch* (HES). Each 100 mL of Hespan contains 6 g of hetastarch and 0.9 g of sodium chloride. The electrolyte concentration is roughly 154 mEq/L each of sodium and chloride. Its efficacy as a volume expander is roughly equivalent to that of albumin 5%.[28] Hespan is excreted via the kidneys. The hydroxyethyl molecules that comprise Hespan tend to be excreted fairly rapidly, but it may take weeks for the starch molecules to be excreted.[28]

INDICATIONS

3 Hespan is indicated primarily as a volume expander in patients who become hypovolemic during elective surgery. Because it also increases the erythrocyte sedimentation rate, it is sometimes indicated in patients who require leukapheresis because it is easier and quicker to remove granulocytes from the blood.

ADVERSE EFFECTS

4 Hespan has antithrombotic effects that are evidenced by diminished platelet aggregation and impairment of the clotting mechanisms. Therefore, patients who receive infusions of Hespan are at risk for coagulopathies and bleeding.[21] There is some evidence that it may increase the risk of bleeding in patients who have had cardiopulmonary bypass surgery.[25] Patients with a known history of bleeding disorders should not receive Hespan.

Hespan may cause anaphylactoid reactions that may be evidenced by dyspnea, wheezing, stridor, chills, urticaria, and laryngeal edema. Some patients with a known allergy to corn also may be allergic to hetastarch. Because it is excreted by the kidneys, Hespan is contraindicated in patients with renal failure.[28]

Dextran

Dextran is a carbohydrate macromolecule that is composed of polymer chains of the glucose molecule. Once infused intravenously, over 50 percent of dextran is excreted by the kidneys, and the remaining amount breaks down slowly into glucose molecules that may be used as a fuel source by the body's cells.

Dextrans that are used as I.V. colloid solutions are either high-molecular-weight dextrans, including 6% Dextran-70, or low-molecular-weight dextrans, including 10% Dextran-40. The weight of these solutions is based on the weight of the dextran molecules, at either 70,000 Da for the high-molecular-weight dextran (Dextran-70) or 40,000 Da for the low-molecular-weight dextran (Dextran-40). Both have roughly equivalent tonicity and osmolality, however. Both solutions are slightly hyperosmotic and hypertonic. They are available in either 0.9% sodium chloride solutions or 5% dextrose solutions.

INDICATIONS

3 Dextrans are indicated for many of the same reasons that other colloids are indicated, that is, for volume expansion for patients in hypovolemic shock or at risk for hypovolemic shock. In addition, Dextran-40 has antithrombotic effects and is particularly indicated in patients at risk for venous thromboemboli formation.[22]

ADVERSE EFFECTS

4 Dextrans carry the greatest relative risk for adverse reactions of all colloids. In particular, dextrans are associated with allergic reactions, anaphylactoid reactions, renal failure, and bleeding disorders[21,25] and can interfere with obtaining appropriate blood crossmatching.[25]

Gelatins

Gelatins are also colloids that are composed primarily of carbohydrate molecules. Some examples of gelatins include modified-fluid gelatin and urea-bridged gelatin.

INDICATIONS

3 Indications for use of gelatins overlap those of other colloids, particularly albumin 5%. Because gelatins tend to have a shorter plasma half-life, a shorter duration of volume expansion achieved, and a greater risk profile than albumin 5%, they are not indicated frequently.

ADVERSE EFFECTS

4 Gelatins carry the same relative risk for causing anaphylactoid reactions as Hespan. Urea-based gelatins contain calcium. As such, they may not be infused in conjunction with I.V. transfusions of packed red blood cells or whole blood or inappropriate clotting may occur.[24,25]

Summary

Colloids are effective at expanding intravascular volume. They can be derived from both nonsynthetic and synthetic sources. They have a variety of uses, but their use should not supplant the use of crystalloids and blood component products when indicated.

Quiz

1. Which of the following statements regarding colloids is *false*?

    (a) Colloids are composed of macromolecules and electrolytes.

    (b) Colloids pass readily through capillary and cell membranes.

(c) Colloids are called volume expanders.

(d) Colloids may be derived from either nonsynthetic or synthetic sources.

2. An example of a nonsynthetic colloid includes

   (a) plasma protein fraction.

   (b) Hespan.

   (c) Dextran.

   (d) urea-bridged gelatin.

3. Indications for I.V. infusions of albumin include *all but which* of the following?

   (a) Burn shock

   (b) Liver failure with ascites

   (c) Leukapheresis

   (d) Pancreatitis

4. Plasma protein fraction (PPF) is composed of *all but which* of the following?

   (a) Albumin

   (b) Carbohydrate macromolecules

   (c) Alpha globulin

   (d) Beta globulin

5. Which of the following colloids may cause a problem with obtaining blood crossmatching when it is infused?

   (a) Albumin

   (b) Plasma protein fraction

   (c) Hespan

   (d) Dextran

6. Which of the following colloids carries the greatest risks for adverse reactions?

   (a) Albumin

   (b) Plasma protein fraction

   (c) Hespan

   (d) Dextran

CHAPTER 9

Blood Component Therapy

Learning Objectives

After completing this chapter, the learner will

1. Identify and describe the most common blood components.

2. Discuss indications for transfusion of common blood components.

3. Compare and contrast the characteristics of common blood components that may be transfused.

4. Describe procedures that ensure safe and effective transfusion of blood components.

5. Differentiate clinical manifestations of common transfusion reactions.

6. Describe protocols to treat transfusion reactions.

Key Terms

Erythrocytes	Fibrinogen
Leukocytes	Anemia
Thrombocytes	Leukopenia
Hematopoiesis	Erythropoietin
Complete blood count (CBC)	Granulocyte colony-stimulating factor
Hematocrit	(G-CSF)
Hemoglobin	Thrombopoietin
Plasma	Thrombocytopenia
Plasma proteins	Whole blood
Albumin	Packed red blood cells
Immunoglobulins	Fresh-frozen plasma
Antigens	Cryoprecipitate

Blood Components Defined

1 Blood consists of blood cells and plasma. Blood cells include red blood cells (i.e., **erythrocytes**), white blood cells (i.e., **leukocytes**), and platelets (i.e., **thrombocytes**). **Hematopoiesis** is defined as the generation of new blood cells. All blood cells are derived from pluripotent stem cells that, in turn, differentiate into generations of more clearly differentiated cells under the stimulation of colony-stimulating factors.[29]

The **complete blood count** (**CBC**) is the laboratory test that analyzes concentrations of blood cells in a sample of blood. Normal values from an adult CBC are displayed in Table 9-1. Erythrocytes are the most abundant blood cells. The volume of erythrocytes in a sample of blood is referred to as the **hematocrit**. The normal hematocrit for an adult male is between 39 and 48 percent and for an adult female is between 36 and 45 percent. The **hemoglobin** molecule comprises most of the weight of each erythrocyte. It is the molecule that transports oxygen. The normal concentration of hemoglobin in a sample of blood for an adult male ranges between 13 and 16 g/dL and for an adult female ranges between 12 and 15 g/dL. Thus the numeric value of the hematocrit is approximately three times the numeric value of the hemoglobin. Erythrocytes live for approximately 90–120 days.[29]

Leukocytes are the blood cells responsible for mounting and modulating host immune and inflammatory responses to pathogens and injurious agents. As such,

Table 9-1   Normal Adult Values on the Complete Blood Count (CBC)

Component	Value
Hematocrit	
Males	39–48%
Females	36–45%
Hemoglobin	
Males	13–16 g/dL
Females	12–15 g/dL
Red blood cell count	
Males	$4.3–5.7 \times 10^6$ cells/mm^3
Females	$3.8–5.1 \times 10^6$ cells/mm^3
White blood cell count	$4.5–11.0 \times 10^3$ cells/mm^3
Platelets	$150–450 \times 10^3$ cells/mm^3

their levels can change dramatically when the host becomes injured or infected. White blood cells include neutrophils, eosinophils, basophils, monocytes, and lymphocytes. The life span of each of these cells can vary considerably from days to years.[29]

Thrombocytes are not true cells in that they are the mature fragments of megakaryocytes. Thrombocytes are the initiators of the clotting cascade. As such, they are necessary in controlling hemorrhage and in initiating repair of injured tissue. Thrombocytes live for only approximately 9 days.[29]

Plasma is the acellular component of blood. It normally comprises approximately 52–64 percent of the volume of a specimen of adult blood. Over 90 percent of plasma is composed of water. Between 6.5 and 8.0 percent of plasma is comprised of various proteins, called the **plasma proteins**.[29] The most important of these plasma proteins include albumin, the immunoglobulins, and fibrinogen. **Albumin** is the plasma protein that is most important in maintaining intravascular colloidal osmotic pressure (COP). It is also important in promoting wound healing. The **immunoglobulins** are antibodies that are preformed by the host's plasma cells, which are derived from B-lymphocytes, to defend the host from foreign substances called **antigens**. **Fibrinogen** is a clotting factor that is important in modulating the common pathway in the coagulation cascade.[30]

In addition to water and the plasma proteins, plasma contains a variety of other substances, including hormones, gases, and electrolytes. Calcium is an electrolyte found in plasma that also functions as a clotting factor (i.e., factor IV).[30]

It is possible to replace deficiencies in virtually any of these previously identified blood components through intravenous transfusion. These blood components may be taken from human donors (i.e., *allogeneic*) or from the original host to store and transfuse back to the host in times of need (i.e., *autologous*). The most common of these blood components available for transfusion will be discussed in the following sections.

SPEED BUMP

Donated blood components are referred to as _____ blood components, whereas blood components withdrawn from the host with the intent to transfuse back to the host in times of need are referred to as _____ blood components.

In general, indications for transfusion of any blood components are more restrictive than they were 25 years ago. These restrictions have been generated in part by recent pharmacologic developments that use recombinant genetic engineering. For instance, it is now possible to administer a variety of recombinantly manufactured colony-stimulating factors to patients with chronic diseases that result in low erythrocyte counts (i.e., **anemia**) or low leukocyte counts (i.e., **leukopenia**). These pharmacologic products include recombinant **erythropoietin** (i.e., epoetin [Epogen, Procrit]) to treat anemia[31] and recombinant **granulocyte colony-stimulating factor (G-CSF)** (i.e., pegfilgrastim [Neulasta]) to treat leukopenia. Clinical research is now aimed at developing a safe and effective recombinant **thrombopoietin,** a colony-stimulating factor that increases the production of platelets to treat low platelet counts, or **thrombocytopenia.**

In addition to these pharmacologic advances, there is now a better understanding that transfusions have adverse effects on host immunity, which also has had the effect of restricting their indications. For instance, human immunodeficiency virus (HIV) and hepatitis B and C viruses were transfused to numerous unsuspecting patients along with their blood components in the 1980s. Sophisticated screening tests thwarted the transmission of these viruses in later years, but within the past few years, West Nile virus, cytomegalovirus (CMV), and the Creutzfeldt-Jakob prion were transmitted to patients receiving blood transfusions.[32] In addition to transmitting viruses and other pathogens, it is now believed that transfusion of allogeneic blood components has both short- and long-term adverse effects on host immunocompetence.[32,33] Patients who receive blood components may be at increased risk for viral infections, bacterial infections, acute lung injury, recurrence of cancers that were in remission, and development of autoimmune disorders later in life.[34]

Types of Blood Components

It was noted in the preceding section that it is possible to transfuse virtually any blood component to patients. While this is possible, the risks associated with transfusing some of these components may outweigh the potential benefits. For instance, there are very few indications that support transfusing white blood cells. Table 9-2 lists the most commonly transfused blood components, the approximate intravenous volume that is infused with each respective unit that is transfused, and their respective indications.

Table 9-2   Commonly Prescribed Blood Components

Blood Component	Approximate Volume	Indications
Whole blood	500 mL/unit	Hemorrhage Anemia with risk of cardiovascular impairment (e.g., myocardial ischemia)
PRBCs	250 mLs/unit	Same as indications for whole blood; generally preferred as first-line therapy
FFP	200 mLs/unit	Rapid reversal of anticoagulant effects of warfarin (Coumadin) Nonspecific replacement of clotting factor deficiencies from acute coagulopathies or liver disease
Platelets	50 mL/unit	Symptomatic thrombocytopenia Platelet count < 10,000/mm^3
Factor VIII	10 mL/unit (after reconstitution)	Hemorrhage or injury associated with hemophilia A Prophylaxis prior to surgery in patients with hemophilia A Hemorrhage associated with von Willebrand disease that is unresponsive to DDAVP
Factor IX	10 mL/unit (after reconstitution)	Hemorrhage associated with hemophilia B (Christmas disease) Prophylaxis prior to surgery in patients with hemophilia B (Christmas disease)
Cryoprecipitate	10 mL/unit	Hemorrhage with hypofibrinogemia or factor XIII deficiency Factor VIII unavailable for treatment of hemophilia A or von Willebrand disease

It was noted in the preceding section that transfusing allogeneic blood components carries significant health risks. The likelihood of experiencing a transfusion-related adverse event increases if a blood component is stored improperly or is used past its expiration date. For instance, a unit of whole blood or packed red blood cells may be stored only for up to 42 days, generally speaking.[35] It is hoped that results from clinical research will one day yield safe and effective blood component substitutes so that these dual problems of host-insulted immunity and product storage may be thwarted. Thus far this quest has not been realized.

WHOLE BLOOD

As its name implies, **whole blood** is plasma and blood cells stored together in their normal state with an added anticoagulant such as citrate and preservatives that may include phosphate, dextrose, adenine, and manitol.[35–37] The rule of thumb is that each unit of whole blood infused should increase the hemoglobin by 1 mg/dL and the hematocrit by 3 percent. Indications for transfusing whole blood include hemorrhage or severe anemia. In years past, any patient with a hemoglobin level of less than 10 g/dL or a hematocrit of less than 30 percent could expect to be a candidate for blood transfusion. Now indications for blood transfusions are more restrictive. Patients who are hemodynamically unstable because of acute blood loss or who are otherwise anemic and at risk of myocardial ischemia are considered transfusion candidates.[33,34] Other anemic patients may be transfused only after a careful assessment of potential transfusion-related risks and benefits is made.

Donated blood is rarely stored as whole blood; rather, it tends to be fractionated into component parts and stored as such.[35] As most donated blood is fractionated, very few patients who are candidates for blood transfusions receive whole blood; rather, they tend to receive transfusions of packed red blood cells (PRBCs; see following section). Autologous blood (i.e., autotransfused blood) commonly is stored as whole blood. Therefore, patients who receive their own previously stored blood tend to receive whole blood, although autologous blood may be fractionated into components if indicated.[35]

Autotransfusion

Autotransfusions (i.e., autologous transfusions) are classified by the methods that describe their withdrawal. These include preoperative autologous blood donation (PABD), acute normovolemic hemodilution (ANH), intraoperative blood salvage (IBS), and postoperative blood salvage (PBS).[37] PABD is storage of autologous blood in advance of surgery that could result in blood loss. So that the patient has sufficient time to manufacture new erythrocytes and thus has a lesser likelihood of being anemic from withdrawal of blood, the blood generally is withdrawn and stored for approximately 4–6 weeks prior to surgery. Blood stored longer than 6 weeks may not maintain its stability. The patient must be healthy at the time that the blood is withdrawn and free of fever or suspected infections.[37]

ANH requires that 1–2 units of the patient's blood is withdrawn and replaced with a matching volume of intravenous crystalloids or colloids in the operating room immediately prior to surgery. The withdrawn blood is reinfused at the end of the surgical case, resulting in less overall surgical blood loss.[37] IBS is similar to ANH in that blood is both lost and then reinfused into the patient while the patient is in the operating room. However, IBS uses blood that is lost during the surgery from the operative site that is then collected and reinfused directly to the patient.[37] PBS reinfuses blood lost from drains and chest tubes back into the postoperative patient.[37]

PACKED RED BLOOD CELLS

Units of **packed red blood cells** (PRBCs) contain the same blood components as whole blood without most of the plasma. Donated blood is centrifuged so that the plasma and the blood cells are separated. As a result, 1 unit of PRBCs contains the same number of erythrocytes, leukocytes, and platelets as 1 unit of whole blood minus most of the plasma. PRBCs generally contain the same anticoagulants and preservatives as whole blood. The indications for transfusing PRBCs mirror those of whole blood, and they generally are used as first-line therapy for allogeneic transfusions because they tend to be more readily available in blood banks than whole blood. Transfusing 1 unit of PRBCs generally will increase the hemoglobin by 1 mg/dL and the hematocrit by 3 percent, as will transfusing 1 unit of whole blood. Although the shelf life of a unit of PRBCs is only approximately 42 days, there are methods that may extend its usefulness, such as biochemical rejuvenation or freezing, as needed if the supply of PRBCs is low.[35]

SPEED BUMP

Donated centrifuged blood that contains erythrocytes, leukocytes, platelets, little plasma, and an anticoagulant and preservatives is referred to as _____

_____.

Modified Packed Red Blood Cells

Patients at increased risk for transfusion-related reactions may need to have their blood units specially prepared or modified. Modified PRBCs may be irradiated, washed, leukocyte-reduced, or specially screened for cytomegalovirus (CMV).

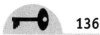

Packets of modified PRBCs are not only specially prepared, but they are also tagged as such and typically are prepared and distributed in donut-shaped intravenous bags in order to make it visually apparent that they have been modified.[35,38]

PRBCs are irradiated with gamma rays to inactivate donor lymphocytes that can cause graft-versus-host disease (GVHD). Patients who are at risk for transfusion-related GVHD and for whom irradiated PRBCs are indicated include those who have had bone marrow transplants and stem cell transplants and those with Hodgkins or non-Hodgkins lymphoma. In addition, patients who receive donated blood from family members are at increased risk for transfusion-associated GVHD for reasons that are not entirely clear. As a consequence, blood donated for use among family members should be irradiated prophylactically prior to administration.[38]

PRBCs are washed in sterile saline to remove plasma proteins and cellular debris that are commonly implicated in transfusion-related allergic reactions. Washing of PRBCs is indicated for patients who have had a previous allergic reaction to a blood component.[38] Leukocytes may be reduced from PRBCs through filtering and other methods for patients who have had a previous febrile nonhemolytic (FNH) reaction to blood transfusions. Patients who have had multiple blood transfusions may be considered candidates for leukocyte-reduced PRBCs, also referred to as *leukocyte-poor PRBCs,* to prevent a febrile reaction from occurring.[38]

PRBCs may be specially screened for CMV, a virus that is commonly carried in a dormant state by many adults. However, patients who are either immunosuppressed (e.g., patients with active neoplasms or patients who have received organ transplants) or who have immature immune systems (e.g., infants younger than 4 weeks of age) and who have not been exposed previously to CMV are at risk for CMV-related sepsis. Therefore, these patients should receive PRBCs that have been screened and deemed clear of CMV.[38]

FRESH-FROZEN PLASMA

Fresh-frozen plasma (FFP) is the fractionated plasma portion of a unit of donated blood that is centrifuged until it contains no erythrocytes, leukocytes, or platelets. FFP may be stored safely in its frozen state for at least 1 year. Once thawed, it must be administered within 6–24 hours. FFP contains many important clotting factors, including factor V, factor VIII, and fibrinogen. Because it is rich in clotting factors, the most common indications for transfusion of FFP is to correct acute coagulopathies, including disseminated intravascular coagulation (DIC), to correct clotting deficiencies because of liver disease, and to reverse the effects of the anticoagulant warfarin (Coumadin). Patients who take warfarin and who may require FFP include those whose clotting times are longer than necessary to provide therapeutic anticoagulation efficacy and who are at risk of bleeding and those whose clotting times are considered therapeutic but who must undergo emergency surgery or another interventional procedure that carries a significant risk of bleeding.[35,36]

PLATELETS

Most units of platelets are pooled from multiple donors who are compatible in terms of blood type (e.g., type A, type B, type AB, and type O) and Rhesus factor (Rh factor). These pooled platelets are centrifuged from donated blood and contain few erythrocytes and leukocytes and little plasma. Transfusions of platelets are indicated for patients who are thrombocytopenic with platelet counts less than 20,000/mm^3 and who are either bleeding or considered at risk of bleeding (e.g., patients who are scheduled to have surgery) or for patients who are severely thrombocytopenic with platelet counts less than 10,000/mm^3. Each unit of platelets transfused will result in a platelet count that is increased by approximately 5000/mm^3. Transfusing platelets to patients with consumptive thrombocytopenic conditions, including idiopathic thrombocytopenia purpura (ITP) and DIC, is controversial.[35,36]

Patients who require repeated transfusions of platelets run the risk of alloimmunization from repeated exposure to a variety of different antigens that are present on both leukocytes and platelets. Alloimmunization can cause either FNH reactions (see the section on transfusion reactions below) or can result in accelerated consumption and death of the transfused platelets. These donor antigens that can cause recipient alloimmunization are collectively referred to as *human leukocyte antigens* (HLAs), although they are present on many cells other than leukocytes. The risk of alloimmunization can be decreased if the recipient's immune system comes into contact with fewer HLAs. This can be accomplished by exposing the recipient's immune system to only one donor's HLAs rather than several donors' HLAs each time the recipient is transfused. Hence single-donor units of platelets, which are derived by plasmapheresis, may be indicated for these patients.[35]

ALBUMIN AND PLASMA PROTEIN FRACTION

Albumin 5%, albumin 25%, and plasma protein fraction (PPF) are derived from pooled human plasma. Their physiologic characteristics, guidelines for administration, indications for use, and adverse effects are discussed in Chapter 8.

IMMUNOGLOBULINS

It was noted earlier that immunoglobulins are antibodies formed by plasma cells to fight antigens. Antigens may be foreign cells, foreign molecules, or pathogens. Once formed by plasma cells, readily detectable levels of some immunoglobulins may remain in the plasma for years. Thus it is possible to plasmapharese preformed immunoglobulins from donated blood. Plasmapharesed immunoglobulin then is pooled together from multiple donors and administered to patients exposed to a specific antigen to boost the patients' immune systems by conferring passive immunity. Immunoglobulins are administered most commonly to Rh-negative women of childbearing years who have been exposed to Rh-positive blood (i.e., Rh(D) immune globulin or RhIG [RhoGAM]) and to patients who have been exposed to hepatitis B (i.e., hepatitis B immune globulin [HBIG]), rabies (i.e., rabies immune globulin [RIG]), tetanus (tetanus immune globulin [TIG]), or varicella (chickenpox) (varicella-zoster immune globulin [VZIG]). In most instances, immunoglobulins are administered in one dose intramuscularly.[35,36]

CLOTTING FACTORS AND CRYOPRECIPITATE

Transfusions of FFP are indicated for patients with general deficiencies in clotting factors. Some patients have specific clotting factor deficiencies that are present most commonly because of an inherited disorder. When these patients become injured or bleed, administering the deficient or absent clotting factor is indicated to promote clot formation, hemostasis, and wound healing.

Cryoprecipitate is obtained from centrifuging slowly thawed plasma and removing proteinaceous clotting factors, including the factor VIII complex (i.e., including factor VIII : C and von Willebrand factor), factor XIII, fibronectin, and fibrinogen. Because it is the only source of commercially available fibrinogen, cryoprecipitate is indicated for use in patients with a primary hypofibrinogemic disorder who are bleeding or at risk of bleeding. It also may be indicated for treating patients who are bleeding or at risk of bleeding who have a primary deficiency of factor XIII or a primary deficiency of factor VIII (e.g., hemophilia A, von Willebrand disease) if factor VIII complex is not available.[35,36] Factor VIII complex concentrate is indicated as a more specific first-line treatment for patients with hemophilia A who are bleeding or injured. It is also indicated for patients with von Willebrand disease who are unresponsive to the first-line effects of desmopressin acetate (DDAVP).[35,36] Factor IX complex concentrate (i.e., prothrombin complex, including Christmas factor) is indicated for treating bleeding or injury in patients with a primary deficiency of factor IX (i.e., hemophilia B or Christmas disease).[35,36]

Procedures for Blood Transfusion ₄

BLOOD TYPES AND COMPATIBILITY

The blood type of recipients must be verified as compatible with the blood type of donated blood prior to transfusion to prevent a potentially life-threatening acute hemolytic reaction (see the following section, which describes this type of transfusion reaction and its treatment). This type of verification is essential whenever whole blood and PRBCs are transfused and preferred when FFP, platelets, and cryoprecipitate are transfused.[35–37]

Blood type refers to key antigens found on the surface of the erythrocytes. These antigens are type A, type B, or the inactive antigen H. The inactive antigen H is referred to as *type O*. These antigens exist in pairs, with one of each conferred genetically by each person's biological mother and father. Therefore, there are six different possible permutations of pairs (i.e., phenotypes). Since A and B are equally dominant, and since O is inactive and therefore recessive, there are four possible expressed blood types (i.e., genotypes). Each possible combination of blood type phenotype and genotype includes the following:

- *AA phenotype:* A genotype with type A blood.
- *AO phenotype:* A genotype with type A blood.
- *BB phenotype:* B genotype with type B blood.
- *BO phenotype:* B genotype with type B blood.
- *AB phenotype:* AB phenotype with type AB blood.
- *OO phenotype:* O genotype with type O blood.[35–37]

Because type O blood contains no active antigens on the surface of its erythrocytes, it can be donated to patients with any blood type without causing a hemolytic reaction. Therefore, patients with type O blood are sometimes referred to as *universal donors*. Conversely, patients with type O blood cannot receive allogeneic blood of any other blood type but O because any type of active erythrocyte antigen would be identified by their plasma cells as foreign, and they would suffer an acute hemolytic reaction. On the other hand, the plasma cells for patients with type AB blood are primed to recognize either A or B antigen types as native to them. Therefore, these patients are referred to as *universal recipients* in that they can receive any type of blood and not suffer an acute hemolytic reaction. By the same token, however, they may donate blood only to patients with type AB blood.[35–37]

An additional important antigen found on the surface of erythrocytes is antigen D. This antigen is referred to as the *rhesus factor* (Rh factor). If it is present, it is

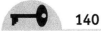

noted as Rh positive. Patients whose erythrocytes do not have the Rh factor are referred to as *Rh negative*. Patients may have any of the four blood types and also be Rh positive or negative. Patients with Rh-positive blood may receive allogeneic blood of an appropriately compatible type that is either Rh positive or Rh negative. However, patients with Rh-negative blood generally should receive only appropriate blood types of Rh-negative blood, or they could form antibodies to the Rh factor that could cause problems with either subsequent transfusions later in life or, in the cases of pregnant Rh-negative women, acute hemolytic reactions in their neonates.[35–37]

INTRAVENOUS DELIVERY SYSTEM

Blood components are stored in blood banks under conditions that maintain the safety and quality of the products as dictated by policies and guidelines advocated by the American Association of Blood Banks (AABB). Prior to obtaining prescribed blood products from the blood bank, the nurse should ensure that the patient has a patent intravenous (I.V.) line in place that can deliver the blood component that is ordered safely and effectively. This is important because transfusions of whole blood or PRBCs must commence within 30 minutes after they are obtained from the blood bank, or they must be returned to the blood bank and not used. Other blood components have similar time restrictions. It is preferred that the venous access catheter be 18 gauge or less, although a 20-gauge catheter may be effective. Both peripheral and central venous access sites are acceptable to transfuse blood components. The I.V. line cannot be used for any other purposes during the blood transfusion, however. If the patient does not have a patent I.V. line, does not have an I.V. line with at least a 20-gauge venous access catheter, or does not have an I.V. line that can be used only for the blood transfusion, then an I.V. line must be started that can accommodate these criteria. In addition to this, the nurse must verify that the patient's informed consent was obtained. Other equipment that should be gathered before the blood component unit is obtained include the following:

- A sterile single-use blood administration set with filter (Fig. 9-1)
- I.V. bag of 0.9% saline to use as the only compatible flush solution
- Equipment for taking vital signs, including stethoscope, blood pressure cuff, and thermometer

Any connectors between I.V. lines must be of the Luer-lock type, according to the *Standards of Practice* promulgated by the Infusion Nurses Society.[6] Additional equipment that might be used could include blood warmers, pressure devices such as pressure bags or fast infusers, and specialized filters. Blood components that are

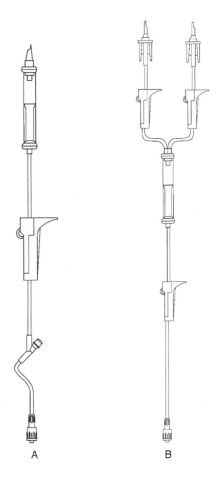

A   B

Figure 9-1 Blood administration sets. *A.* One roller clamp, drip chamber with 170-μm blood filter, and distal-end injection port. *B.* Y-type with three roller clamps, drip chamber with 170-μm blood filter, and distal-end injection port. (Courtesy of B. Braun, Products Catalog, 2005.)

transfused relatively quickly may need to be warmed so that the patient does not become hypothermic. The only approved method to warm blood is by using an AABB-approved blood warmer that is properly maintained and deemed reliable by biomedical engineering professionals at the sponsoring institution. Other methods for warming blood, including immersion of the bag in warmed water, microwaves, etc., are forbidden. If pressure devices or fast infusers are used, similarly they must be AABB-approved devices that have a pressure gauge and exert uniform pressure against all parts of the blood component bag. Leukocyte and microaggregate filters also must meet industry safety and quality standards if they are prescribed.[6]

VERIFICATION PROCEDURES

Prior to initiating a transfusion of a prescribed blood component, the nurse verifies the appropriateness of the order.[6] The nurse must verify that informed consent for transfusion has been obtained and that the patient understands the indications for the transfusion, its associated risks and benefits, and whether there might be any alternatives to transfusion.[35,39] Asking patients whether or not they have ever had prior blood transfusions and, if so, whether they had any type of adverse reaction to the transfusion is helpful. Patients who belong to a Jehovah's Witness congregation may refuse transfusion based on their religious beliefs, and this decision must be respected and documented per agency or hospital protocols.[40] After these procedures, the nurse then takes a baseline set of vital signs, including the patient's temperature, blood pressure, heart rate, and respiratory rate, and records these data in the patient's record. It is good practice for the nurse to listen to the patient's baseline heart and lung sounds to determine if there are any extra heart sounds, murmurs, crackles, or wheezes.

Both the AABB and the Joint Commission on Accreditation of Health Care Organizations (JCAHO) mandate that at least two identifiers be used to verify that the right patient is receiving the right blood component.[39] The patient's full name typically is one of these identifiers and is present on the blood component product bag and the patient's identification bag. The patient also should be asked to state his or her full name. Other identifiers may include the patient's date of birth or Social Security Number or the hospital identification number. The patient's hospital room number is not considered an appropriate identifier.[6] The current *Standards of Practice* for the Infusion Nurses Society further specifies that two licensed professionals must verify that the appropriate blood component is matched to the appropriate patient.[6]

ADMINISTRATION PROCEDURES

Once it is determined that the right patient is receiving the right blood component at the right time and for the right reason, the transfusion may be initiated.[39] The I.V. line is flushed with 0.9% normal saline, and the blood component then is flushed into the line at a slow initial infusion rate. The most serious, life-threatening transfusion reactions tend to occur within the first 15 minutes of transfusion. Therefore, most blood transfusions begin slowly, and the patient is monitored carefully for the first 15 minutes after the beginning of therapy. For patients who are in hemorrhagic shock, this protocol is not followed because quick replacement of lost blood supersedes this safety protocol. Many agencies require that the nurse assess the patient's vital signs and temperature once every 5 minutes for the first 15 minutes and then at lengthier intervals as the transfusion continues. Most transfusions should be either completed or discontinued within 4 hours. If the patient requires several units of the same blood component, then the same protocols are repeated for each subsequent transfusion, and the unit administration setup is changed so that a new, sterile blood administration setup is used.[6,37]

MONITORING FOR TRANSFUSION REACTIONS 5

The nurse must assess the patient carefully for clinical manifestations of transfusion reactions during transfusion of blood components. The most common transfusion reactions are discussed in the following sections. These may include acute hemolytic reaction, febrile nonhemolytic reaction, transfusion-related acute lung injury, allergic reaction, volume overload, and bacteremia.

Acute Hemolytic Reaction

An acute hemolytic reaction occurs when a patient is transfused with the wrong blood type. Clinical manifestations tend to occur very quickly, within 5–15 minutes after the transfusion commences. These include the following:

- Chills
- Fever
- Low back pain
- Tachypnea
- Tachycardia
- Hypotension
- Pain and flushing at the infusion site

When the wrong type of blood component is transfused, the transfused erythrocytes are recognized by the recipient's plasma cells as foreign, and host antibodies attack these cells, causing rapid erythrocyte destruction or hemolysis. By-products of rapid erythrocyte destruction clog the renal tubules, resulting in low back pain, hematuria, and acute renal failure. In addition, because the recipient's immune system mounts an acute systemic response, the patient mounts a fever and exhibits signs consistent with shock.[36,37]

Febrile Nonhemolytic Reaction

Febrile nonhemolytic (FNH) reactions occur when the recipient's plasma cells form antibodies to HLAs found on transfused leukocytes or platelets. The likelihood that these reactions will occur increases with lengthier transfusion times and with repeated blood transfusions. Therefore, guidelines for transfusing whole blood or PRBCs specify that each unit infuse within 4 hours to decrease the likelihood that FNH reactions occur. Patients with a prior history of an FNH reaction or who are at increased risk for an FNH reaction because they have had multiple transfusions may be candidates for prophylactic transfusions of leukocyte-reduced PRBCs. In addition, these patients may benefit if an antipyretic such as acetaminophen is administered immediately prior to commencement of the transfusion.[36,37]

Clinical manifestations of an FNH reaction may include the following:

- Chills
- Fever
- Headache
- Myalgias
- Nausea
- Chest pain[36,37]

Transfusion-Related Acute Lung Injury

The pathophysiologic mechanism responsible for transfusion-related acute lung injury (TRALI) is similar to that found in FNH reactions in that the recipient's immune system forms antibodies to allogeneically donated leukocytes. For reasons that are not entirely clear, however, the response in TRALI tends to be much quicker than that found in FNH reactions and tends to cause acute respiratory failure followed by a type of acute respiratory distress syndrome. These patients tend to respond well to early recognition, aggressive management of acute respiratory failure, and I.V. administration of corticosteroids.[35-37]

Allergic Reactions

Most allergic reactions to allogeneically transfused blood are mild and occur as a result of immunoglobulin E (IgE)–regulated sensitivity to the donated blood's plasma proteins. This type of reaction typically is delayed and occurs either toward the end of the transfusion or within a couple of hours after the transfusion is completed. Clinical manifestations include

- Flushing
- Urticaria (i.e., hives)
- Itching, particularly of the palms of the hands and soles of the feet

Patients with a prior history of a variety of other allergies are particularly susceptible to this type of urticarial reaction to a blood transfusion. Patients with known prior histories of urticarial allergic reactions to blood transfusions may benefit from administration of diphenhydramine (Benadryl) immediately prior to commencement of subsequent transfusions to mitigate these allergic manifestations.[36,37]

Infrequently, allergic reactions to allogeneically transfused blood can be IgE-mediated and thus exhibit as an anaphylactic type of reaction. This type of reaction typically occurs early during the first few minutes of the transfusion, and the patient rapidly deteriorates into anaphylactic shock unless rapid interventions are taken. These clinical manifestions include the same signs and symptoms that are consistent with an allergic reaction plus the following:

- Wheezing with respiratory distress, followed by stridor and laryngospasms
- Nausea, abdominal pains, severe cramping
- Tachycardia
- Hypotension with narrowed pulse pressure[36,37]

Circulatory Overload

Patients with a history of heart failure or those at risk of heart failure may not be able to handle rapid I.V. infusion of blood components and may exhibit clinical manifestations of acute heart failure or circulatory overload. Thus it is important that the nurse monitor and document the patient's baseline vital signs and assess and document the patient's baseline heart and lung sounds before transfusions are begun. These baseline data may be compared with data derived during and after transfusion to determine whether or not the patient is suffering from circulatory overload or acute heart failure. Clinical manifestations consistent with circulatory overload include the following:

- Angina
- Dyspnea
- Tachycardia
- Tachypnea
- Hypotension
- Bibasilar crackles
- Coughing
- Hemoptysis
- S_3
- Oliguria

Patients with a known history of heart failure and who are considered at risk for circulatory overload may benefit from having their blood components administered more slowly. In some instances, it may be advisable to request that blood bank professionals prepare "split packs" of PRBCs so that patients with heart failure do not receive entire units of blood products within 4-hour time limits. Other prophylactic interventions may revolve around administering prophylactic I.V. loop diuretics to these patients so that they can receive maximum benefits of myocardial oxygenation from transfused blood cells while overall increases in blood volume are minimized, thus diminishing myocardial workload and the likelihood of circulatory overload.

Bacteremia and Sepsis

Contamination of the transfused blood component with pathogens, most commonly bacteria, can cause blood-borne bacterial infections (i.e., bacteremia) and systemic infection (i.e., sepsis). This can be prevented through administering the blood components within the specified time limits, by maintaining the sterility of the I.V. administration setup with Luer-lock connections, and by changing I.V. blood administration sets every 4 hours or with the administration of each new blood component unit. In addition, I.V. administration sets should be changed anytime that contamination is suspected.[6] Clinical manifestations of bacteremia and sepsis may vary widely from fever and chills to manifestations that are consistent with septic shock.[35–37]

General Protocols for Treating Transfusion Reactions [6]

Whenever any type of transfusion reaction is suspected, there are some general protocols that must be instituted. First of all, if the patient is still receiving the transfusion, it must be stopped immediately. The physician is notified, and the exact clinical manifestations that the patient exhibits are reported and documented carefully. The patient identification protocol is repeated to ensure that the patient received the right blood component product.[35,39] The I.V. access line is flushed with 0.9% sterile saline and kept patent in the event that emergent I.V. push medications are indicated or in case the patient requires emergent fluid volume resuscitation. Blood and urine specimens are obtained and sent to the blood bank for analysis, along with the original blood component infusion set and bag with its remaining blood component contents.[35,39]

SPEED BUMP

If a patient is suspected of exhibiting manifestations of any type of transfusion reaction, the first treatment intervention that must be instituted is _____ _____.

Summary

Transfusions of specific blood components may be indicated to correct acute life-threatening blood component deficiencies. Almost any major blood component may be transfused. The advent of recombinant pharmacologic blood component colony-stimulating factors has supplanted some indications for blood transfusion. In addition, a heightened awareness that transfusion with blood components can have deleterious short- and long-term effects on immune function has further limited indications for blood transfusions. Nurses administering transfusions must thoroughly understand the policies and protocols that govern safe and effective delivery of transfusions. In addition, they must be adept at recognizing transfusion reactions when they occur and intervening quickly to prevent further morbidity and mortality.

Quiz

1 A normal adult male hemoglobin level is

   (a) 15 g/dL.

   (b) 45 percent.

   (c) 12 g/dL.

   (d) 5.0×10^6 cells/mm^3.

2. Leukopenia may be treated safely and effectively with

   (a) leukocyte transfusions.

   (b) whole blood transfusions.

   (c) recombinant granulocyte colony-stimulating factor (G-CSF).

   (d) recombinant erythropoietin.

3. The expiration date for whole blood or packed red blood cells is approximately

   (a) 30 minutes after it is donated.

   (b) 9 days after it is donated.

   (c) 30 days after it is donated.

   (d) 42 days after it is donated.

4. Each unit of packed red blood cells that is transfused should increase the hematocrit by

   (a) 1 percent.

   (b) 3 percent.

   (c) 5 percent.

   (d) 10 percent.

5. The method of autotransfusion that uses blood that is withdrawn from the patient 4–6 months preoperatively and stored in case the patient requires blood transfusions postoperatively is

   (a) preoperative autologous blood donation (PABD).

   (b) acute normovolemic hemodilution (ANH).

   (c) intraoperative blood salvage (IBS).

   (d) postoperative blood salvage (PBS).

6. Which of the following types of modified units of packed red blood cells (PRBCs) may be indicated for patients with a history of febrile nonhemolytic reactions?

   (a) Irradiated

   (b) Washed

   (c) Leukoctye-reduced

   (d) CMV screened

7. Transfusions of platelets are indicated for

   (a) all patients who are thrombocytopenic (i.e., have lower than normal platelet counts).

   (b) all patients with bleeding disorders or coagulopathies.

   (c) all patients with platelet counts of less than $10,000/mm^3$.

   (d) all patients with consumptive platelet disorders such as idiopathic thrombocytopenia purpura (ITP).

8. Transfusions of fresh-frozen plasma (FFP) are indicated for

   (a) patients with hemophilia A and bleeding or injury.

   (b) patients with hemophilia B and bleeding or injury.

(c) patients with von Willebrand disease with bleeding and injury.

(d) patients receiving warfarin (Coumadin) who require quick reversal of its anticoagulation effects.

9. A patient with an AO phenotype will have which blood type?

(a) Type A

(b) Type B

(c) Type AB

(d) Type O

10. Patients with which blood type can receive transfusions of type A, type B, and type O blood?

(a) Type A

(b) Type B

(c) Type AB

(d) Type O

11. Which patients with Rh-negative blood type must receive transfusions of Rh-negative blood types?

(a) All patients who are Rh-negative

(b) Elderly men

(c) Elderly women

(d) Women of childbearing years

12. Which of the following must be verified prior to commencing a transfusion?

(a) Patient's informed consent

(b) Physician's order

(c) Two unique patient identifiers that match and are found on both the blood component and the patient

(d) All of the above

13. The transfusion reaction that is life-threatening and tends to manifest quickly when patients are transfused with the wrong blood type is a(an)

(a) acute hemolytic reaction.

(b) febrile nonhemolytic reaction.

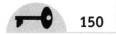

(c) transfusion-related acute lung injury.

(d) allergic reaction.

14. The transfusion reaction that tends to occur with lengthier transfusion times and/or with repeated blood transfusions is a(an)

(a) acute hemolytic reaction.

(b) febrile nonhemolytic reaction.

(c) transfusion-related acute lung injury.

(d) allergic reaction.

15. Intravenous access lines for blood transfusions

(a) may be flushed only with sterile water.

(b) may use only 16-gauge access catheters.

(c) may be used for access of I.V. push diuretics as needed.

(d) must use secure Luer-lock connections as appropriate.

CHAPTER 10

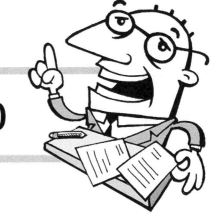

Parenteral Nutrition Therapy

Learning Objectives

After completing this chapter, the learner will

1. Identify indications for parenteral nutrition therapy.

2. Compare and contrast the composition of commonly prescribed parenteral nutrition solutions.

3. Discuss methods for delivery of parenteral nutrition solutions.

4. Describe methods that ensure safe initiation, maintenance, and discontinuation of parenteral nutrition infusions.

5. Identify common short- and long-term complications associated with parenteral nutrition therapy.

Key Terms

Parenteral nutrition	Total parenteral nutrition
Hyperalimentation	Total nutrient admixture
Enteral nutrition	Fat emulsions

Parenteral Nutrition Defined

Parenteral nutrition (PN) refers to the delivery of nutrients into a central or peripheral vein by an intravenous (I.V.) delivery system that is sometimes also called **hyperalimentation**. PN is administered either as a sole source of nutrition or to supplement enteral feedings. **Enteral nutrition** refers to the delivery of nutrients through the gastrointestinal tract, either naturally or by using feeding tubes that deliver nutrients into the stomach, duodenum, or jejunum. Delivering nutrients by the enteral route is preferred to delivering nutrients by the parenteral route whenever possible because when the gastrointestinal tract is not used, villous atrophy occurs, and the gastrointestinal tract's competency at digesting and metabolizing nutrients in the future becomes compromised.

1 In some instances, it may not be possible to meet patients' total nutritional needs through either natural means or administering gastric, duodenal, or jejunal tube feedings. These patients include those who cannot completely absorb nutrients because of short bowel syndrome, for instance. Not administering nutrients sufficient to meet daily caloric needs can lead to hypoalbuminemia and negative nitrogen balance, which can lead to loss of skeletal muscle mass and cachexia, poor wound healing, and diminished immunocompetence. Thus these patients may require the delivery of additional nutrients parenterally.

In some instances, patients are unable to ingest or absorb any nutrients enterally. These patients must have their nutritional requirements met completely through nutrients delivered by a parenteral route. Examples of patients who would require this include those patients who have gastrointestinal fistulas and intestinal obstructions.[41]

SPEED BUMP

_____ *refers to the delivery of nutrients into a central or peripheral vein by an I.V. delivery system.*

Types of Parenteral Nutrition

PN solutions are admixed individually in pharmacies using aseptic techniques under laminar flow hoods.[6] The formula used to admix any PN solution is based on the individual patient's calculated fluid, electrolyte, and caloric requirements. In tandem with these considerations, the patient's specific metabolic needs that can affect fluid, electrolyte, micronutrient, and macronutrient requirements are taken into account to prepare the most nutritionally complete parenteral solution possible for that patient.

TOTAL PARENTERAL NUTRITION SOLUTIONS

Most PN solutions contain over 30 different components, including water, electrolytes, micronutrients, and macronutrients. The amount of water that should be delivered with PN solutions is approximately 30–35 mL/kg per day.[42] Electrolytes may include the following:

- Sodium, with a recommended daily requirement of 40–50 mEq
- Potassium, with a recommended daily requirement of 30–40 mEq
- Chloride, with a recommended daily requirement of 40–50 mEq
- Phosphate, with a recommended daily requirement of 15–25 mmol
- Magnesium, with a recommended daily requirement of 8–12 mEq
- Calcium, with a recommended daily requirement of 2–5 mEq[43]

Micronutrients include vitamins and trace minerals. The vitamins composition of typical PN solutions includes the following:

- 1 mg vitamin A (retinol)
- 3 mg vitamin B_1 (thiamine)
- 3.6 mg vitamin B_2 (riboflavin)
- 15 mg vitamin B_3 (niacin)
- 4 mg vitamin B_6 (pyridoxine)
- 60 µg vitamin B_7 (biotin)
- 400 µg vitamin B_9 (folic acid)
- 5 µg vitamin B_{12} (cobalamin)
- 100 mg vitamin C (ascorbic acid)
- 5 µg vitamin D (ergocalciferol)
- 10 IU vitamin E (tocopherol)[43]

Patients who are not taking oral anticoagulants (e.g., warfarin [Coumadin]) may be prescribed PN solutions that also contain 1–4 mg/day vitamin K.[42,43] Trace minerals that typically are admixed to PN solutions include zinc, chromium, copper, manganese, and sometimes selenium. Vitamins and trace elements are essential components of PN solutions because they ensure that macronutrients can be metabolized appropriately.[42,43]

Macronutrients added to PN solutions include proteins and carbohydrates and sometimes fats. PN solutions that contain proteins and carbohydrates are sometimes referred to as *2-in-1 PN solutions* or sometimes **total parenteral nutrition (TPN)** solutions. Patients who receive infusions of the 2-in-1 TPN solutions require supplemental parenteral infusions of fat emulsions (see below). PN formulas that contain all three essential macronutrients of proteins, carbohydrates, and fats are sometimes referred to as *3-in-1 PN solutions* or sometimes **total nutrient admixtures (TNAs)**. The following section describes TNAs in more detail.

The amount of proteins and carbohydrates in any 2-in-1 TPN formulas can be highly variable based on the individual patient's calculated needs and metabolic state. The most common carbohydrate source is dextrose, which can range in solution concentrations from 5–70 percent.[43] Glycerol sometimes is also used as an additional source of carbohydrates in TPN solutions. TPN solutions with a dextrose concentration that is greater than 10 percent should be infused through a central venous access site.[42]

Protein is provided by admixing amino acids with the solution at approximately 0.8 g/kg per day. The actual prescribed TPN concentration of protein can vary considerably depending on the patient's metabolic state and ability to metabolize proteins.[42] For instance, patients with acute renal failure may not be able to rid themselves of the nitrogen that is a by-product of amino acid metabolism and can become azotemic. Therefore, these patients typically are prescribed fewer amino acids in their TPN solutions.

TPN solutions are clear yellow in color. Because TPN solutions become unstable when exposed to light and extremes in temperature, they are typically stored in a refrigerator.[44] It is recommended that these bags be removed from the refrigerator 1 hour before they are hung so that a cold solution is not infused into the patient.[6,45] If a TPN I.V. bag is hanging for more than 24 hours, it should be changed because it may become unstable.[44,45] Each bag of TPN solution should be examined closely before it is hung for any evidence of precipitate or particulate matter. If either of these is present, the bag should not be hung and should be returned to the pharmacy. It is possible that TPN solutions can contain precipitate or particulate matter that is not visible. To prevent patients from receiving infused precipitate or particulate matter that can become emboli, TPN I.V. setups should include a 0.2-μm filter.[6]

SPEED BUMP

Parenteral nutrition solutions contain water, electrolytes, micronutrients that include _____ and trace minerals and macronutrients that include proteins, _____, and sometimes fats.

TOTAL NUTRIENT ADMIXTURES

TNAs are not true solutions because they contain fat emulsions in addition to containing amino acids, dextrose, and glycerol in concentrations similar to those found in TPN. TNAs are milky white in appearance because of these added fat emulsions. TNAs behave similarly to TPN solutions when they are exposed to light or temperature extremes and should be treated the same. Before a bag of TNA is hung, it should be examined to ensure that its appearance is uniformly white. If there is any evidence of oil droplets, frothiness, or discoloration, the bag should not be hung but should be returned to the pharmacy.[44]

A disadvantage to using TNAs is that it may not be readily apparent whether or not there is precipitation or particulate matter in the solution. Therefore, TNA I.V. setups always should include a 1.2-μm filter.[6] Advantages to using TNAs rather than TPN solutions and fat emulsions include decreased overall cost, decreased nursing time associated with hanging fewer I.V. infusions, and decreased likelihood of bacteremia from less frequent manipulation of the I.V. access site.[41,44]

FAT EMULSIONS

Fat emulsions must be prescribed as additional supplements for patients who are receiving TPN. Fatty acids contained in **fat emulsions** provide essential nutrients that cannot be obtained through other nutritional sources. Deficiencies in fatty acids can result in poor wound healing and chronic diarrhea.[42] Patients who receive TNAs do not require supplemental fat emulsions because their 3-in-1 formula already contains sufficient concentrations of fatty acids.

Fat emulsions typically are administered in the form of a commercially packaged formula of safflower oil, soybean oil, and egg phospholipids in either a 10% or 20% concentration. These I.V. fat emulsions (IVFEs) typically are packaged in 500-mL bottles with their own special infusion lines that can be administered concomitant with the TPN solution by a Y-connector past the point of the TPN filter. IVFEs typically are infused three times a week over 6- to 12-hour infusion intervals. Prior to administering IVFEs, the nurse should examine the IVFE bottle for any evidence of instability. The solution should appear uniformly milky without any evidence of heterogeneity, oiliness, frothiness, or discoloration. If it is suspected that the solution is unstable, it should be returned to the pharmacy.[42,43]

Patients with a history of allergies to eggs or to safflower or soybean products or oils should not be prescribed IVFEs.[42,43] Some patients without a known allergy to any of these nonetheless may exhibit an immunoglobulin E (IgE)–mediated allergic reaction. These may be exhibited by flushing, urticaria (i.e., hives), and itching, particularly of the palms of the hands or soles of the feet. If the patient exhibits any of these signs during infusion, the infusion must be discontinued immediately and the physician notified. Some patients may exhibit some of these manifestations shortly after the IVFE infusion has finished. The physician should be notified of this event before another IVFE infusion is begun. Any signs or symptoms that suggest that the patient has exhibited an allergic response to the IVFE should be documented in the patient's record.

Methods of Delivering Parenteral Nutrition 3

CONTINUOUS

All acutely ill patients who receive PN have this administered by a continuous I.V. infusion. These patients' total daily fluid, caloric, and nutritional needs are delivered over a continuous 24-hour infusion.

CYCLIC

Patients who receive PN long term and who are outpatients may have their PN delivered over a 12- to 18-hour daily cycle.[46] Patients eligible for this type of cyclic therapy must first evidence physiologic stability on continuous PN, as evidenced by stable blood glucose levels, before the transition can be made to cyclic therapy. Patients who are the best candidates for cyclic I.V. PN are those who can partially meet their nutritional requirements enterally. Advocates of cyclic PN for outpatients assert that these patients have improved quality of life in that they have periodic freedom from being set up to I.V. infusions.[42]

PERIPHERAL AND CENTRAL

Most PN solutions must be infused by central venous access routes. Most TPN and TNA solutions are too hypertonic to be delivered into peripheral veins without quickly causing thrombosis and phlebitis (see Chapter 6 for descriptions of thrombosis and phlebitis and their respective treatments). Central I.V. access sites for infusing

TPN and TNA solutions may include peripherally inserted central catheters (PICCs), nontunneled central catheters, tunneled central catheters, and implanted ports (see Chapter 5 for a comparison of these types of central I.V. access).

PN solutions that contain 10 percent or less of dextrose may be delivered peripherally without incurring heightened risks of thrombosis and phlebitis over the short term. Patients who are candidates for receiving these types of less dextrose-dense solutions by a peripheral access route are those slated to receive PN as supplements to enteral feedings. In general, the anticipated length of peripheral parenteral nutrition (PPN) therapy may not exceed 7 days, or the attendant risks of thrombosis and phlebitis outweigh the benefits of therapy.

SPEED BUMP

Parenteral nutrition solutions that might be infused by peripheral venous access sites contain _____.

Procedures for Administering Parenteral Nutrition

INTRAVENOUS DELIVERY SYSTEM

As noted previously, most PN solutions are infused continuously and by central venous access sites. Although PN solutions may be compatible with some medications, it is generally advocated that TPN and TNA solutions infuse in their own dedicated lines.[6] The less often that these dedicated lines are accessed or manipulated, the lesser is the likelihood that they will become contaminated.

TPN, TNA, and IVFE solutions should be infused using an electronic infusion device or I.V. pump.[6] The prescription for the composition of the TPN, TNA, and/or IVFE solutions and their respective hourly rates of delivery must be made by a physician or advanced-practice clinician with prescriptive authority authorized by the respective governing state board of nursing or medicine. The nurse must verify that the right PN solution is prescribed for the right patient at the right prescriptive dosages and formulations, by the right venous access route, and at the right hourly rate. To verify this, the patient and the TPN or TNA bag must be double-checked prior to initiation of therapy by two professionals with the patient's name and two identifiers that may not include the patient's room number.[6]

Any type of PN must be infused completely within 24 hours after it is hung or it must be discarded because it may become unstable. The I.V. administration sets (e.g., I.V. tubing) must be changed using aseptic technique at least every 72 hours if only TPN is infused. If TNAs or IVFEs are infused, the I.V. delivery sets must be changed every 24 hours.[45]

Compatibility of Pharmacologic Agents

As noted previously, the I.V. line that is used for delivery of TPN or TNA solution should be dedicated to that purpose alone, with the exception of IVFEs, which may be piggybacked into a TPN line.[6] Some medications are commonly admixed with the TPN or TNA solution in their infusion containers or I.V. bags because they are indicated for use in most of these patients and generally are considered compatible with these types of solutions used. These medications include insulin, famotidine (Pepcid), and ranitidine (Zantac).[44] Although these medications are considered compatible with TPN and TNA solutions, they should not be added to TPN or TNA I.V. bags after they have begun to infuse[6] or the hourly dosage rate may be difficult to validate. Any medications that are admixed to TPN or TNA I.V. bags should be highlighted on the labels on the respective PN bags with the admixed dose, the date the medication was added, and the initials of the clinician who admixed the medication in the PN solution.[6]

INITIATING THERAPY

TPN and TNA solutions should be initiated at hourly rates that are slower than those prescribed for the long term. Typical initiation regimens begin at 40–50 mL/h, which is increased each subsequent hour by 25 mL for up to 6 hours until the desired hourly infusion rate is met. At this point, the patient may be maintained at the desired hourly infusion rate on a continuous basis.

MONITORING EFFECTIVENESS OF THERAPY

Patients receiving continuous infusions of TPN or TNA solutions in the acute-care setting should have serum glucose levels assessed every 6 hours for at least 48 hours and then every 24 hours thereafter if glucose levels are normal. Many patients will require continued 6-hour assessments of their blood glucose levels for the long term and will require sliding-scale insulin coverage and/or insulin admixed with their TPN or TNA solution. Other assessments that should be performed on a daily basis include weights, intake and output, and serum electrolytes. Albumin and prealbumin levels should be assessed at least weekly.[42]

MONITORING FOR ADVERSE EVENTS   5

Related to I.V. Access

Patients who receive PN infusions by central I.V. access routes are at risk for the same associated problems of hemothorax, pneumothorax, air embolism, thrombosis, and infection that accompany use of a central venous access device, which were identified in Chapter 5.[42]

Sepsis

Bacteremia and sepsis are common complications associated with the use of PN infusions. This is true partly because most of these solutions use central I.V. access sites with multiple lumens that are accessed numerous times on a daily basis, making them more susceptible to iatrogenic entry of pathogens, and partly because PN solutions are ideal media for the growth of bacterial colonies.

Methods previously identified to diminish the likelihood of sepsis should be employed. In addition, all clinicians should wash their hands prior to touching any TPN, TNA, or IVFE administration set and wear clean gloves. Dressings and lines should be changed at least every 72 hours if they did not infuse any type of fat emulsions (e.g., TPN) and every 24 hours if they were used to deliver fat emulsions (e.g., TNAs and IVFEs). Dressings and administration setups should be also be changed whenever they become contaminated. TPN, TNA, and IVFE solutions should be discarded if they are not fully infused within 24 hours.

Allergic Reactions

Allergic reactions may occur with the infusion of any type of parenteral nutrient but occur most commonly when fat emulsions are introduced, as noted previously in that section.

Fluid and Electrolyte Imbalances

Hyperglycemia is the most common complication associated with administration of PN solutions.[43] If undetected, it can lead to hyperosmolar hyperglycemic nonketotic (HHNK) coma, which can result in life-threatening dehydration. Patients with HHNK coma may manifest blood glucose levels in excess of 600 mg/dL. The excessive serum glucose acts as an osmotic diuretic, and excessive thirst and polyuria are common clinical indicators. This life-threatening syndrome can be treated with administration of I.V. insulin and generous infusions of crystalloids.

HHNK coma can be prevented by monitoring the patient's blood glucose levels periodically as ordered, particularly when PN therapy is being initiated.[47]

Any type of electrolyte imbalance identified previously in Chapter 3 might be exhibited by a patient receiving PN infusions. These may include hypernatremia, hyponatremia, hyperkalemia, hypokalemia, hypercalcemia, hypocalcemia, hyperphosphatemia, hypophosphatemia, hypermagnesemia, and hypomagnesemia.[47] Patients may be treated for these electrolyte disturbances by interventions also described in Chapter 3 or by adjusting electrolyte concentrations in their TPN or TNA solutions.

Hyperglycemia and Hypoglycemia

As noted previously, the most common complication associated with administering TPN or TNA solutions is hyperglycemia.[43,48] This can be prevented by carefully assessing periodic blood glucose levels, particularly when PN is initiated, when its rate of infusion is altered, or when the patient's caloric requirements change because of stress related to disease states or interventions such as surgery. In general, patients who are beginning TPN or TNA infusions should have their blood glucose levels monitored at least every 6 hours and should be provided sliding-scale insulin coverage. For patients whose blood glucose levels are continuously greater than 140 mg/dL or less than 90 mg/dL, blood glucose monitoring may need to occur as frequently as every hour. For patients whose blood glucose levels remain chronically high and who require consistent every-6-hour insulin coverage, insulin may be mixed with the PN solution.[48]

Hypoglycemia may occur if the PN solution is stopped abruptly.[48] This may occur if a PN I.V. bag that is ready to be hung becomes contaminated and cannot be hung because of the heightened risk of bacteremia. The pharmacy must be notified to admix a new sterile I.V. bag of PN solution. In the interim, an I.V. bag of 10% dextrose can be hung at the same hourly rate as the PN solution. This substitute certainly will not provide a complete source of nutrients for the patient but will provide a bridge to therapy that can prevent a life-threatening hypoglycemic reaction from occurring until a new sterile I.V. bag of PN solution is available.

Refeeding Syndrome

Refeeding syndrome describes a systemic response that occurs when nutrients and fluids are administered too suddenly to a patient who has been severely malnourished for a long time. The rapid introduction of electrolytes, vitamins, and macronutrients causes rapid and severe disruption in fluid and electrolyte balance, resulting in heart failure, generalized edema, and acute renal failure. This may be treated by administering diuretic agents and by adjusting the rate and composition of the PN solution. The best prevention of refeeding syndrome is prevention. A patient known to be severely malnourished should be prescribed a low initial PN infusion rate. The rate of infusion then is increased slowly based on continued satisfactory assessment of the patient's fluid and electrolyte status and the satisfactory response of the patient's cardiovascular system to the therapy.[42]

Long-Term Metabolic Complications

Patients who are maintained on PN solutions for the long term may develop a host of idiosyncratic complications. These may include liver failure from hepatic steatosis or steatohepatitis, cholelithiasis and cholestasis, manganese toxicity that is associated with a neurotoxic parkinsonism, and metabolic bone disease.[48] The best treatment of these disorders is prevention—by instituting enteral feedings as soon as reasonably possible and then discontinuing PN therapy. Patients who cannot be fed enterally and must be maintained on PN for weeks or months must be scrutinized closely for their responses to PN therapy because most of these complications are related to overfeeding.[48]

DISCONTINUING THERAPY

Patients who receive PN cannot have their infusions stopped abruptly, or they may exhibit rebound hypoglycemia (see the discussion in the section on hyperglycemia and hypoglycemia above). Rather, these infusions must be diminished gradually so that blood glucose levels are consistently maintained. Patients who were not receiving enteral feedings previously and who are now either beginning to eat or who are gradually being fed enteral tube feedings might have their PN infusions tapered down gradually while their enteral feedings increase gradually until the PN infusions can be stopped safely. Another method to effectively discontinue PN infusions includes discontinuing centrally infused PN infusions while concomitantly introducing peripherally infused 10% dextrose solutions that may, in turn, be changed to 5% dextrose solutions that are then titrated down and eventually discontinued safely.[42,43]

Summary

PN therapy is indicated for patients who cannot receive their complete daily nutritional needs by the enteral route. PN solutions include individually prescribed complex mixtures of water, electrolytes, trace elements, vitamins, amino acids, carbohydrates, and fatty acids. In addition to these, some medications may be added to PN solutions. PN solutions may be administered centrally or peripherally and on a continuous or a cyclic basis, although they are most often administered continuously via a central venous access route. The most common life-threatening complication associated with PN use is hyperglycemia, but many other short- and long-term complications are associated with the use of PN. The nurse must be cognizant of these complications and methods to prevent and treat them in order to deliver optimal care to patients receiving PN infusions.

Quiz

1. For which of the following patients might PN therapy be indicated?

    (a) A patient who has acute pancreatitis

    (b) A patient who has cancer and has lost weight

    (c) A patient who has mouth sores and has difficulty chewing

    (d) A patient with a bowel obstruction

2. Which of the following patients might *not* have vitamin K admixed to his or her TPN solution?

    (a) A patient who is bleeding

    (b) A patient who is prescribed heparin

    (c) A patient who is prescribed warfarin (Coumadin)

    (d) A patient who is hyperkalemic

3. Which of the following PN formulas contains amino acids, carbohydrates, and fatty acids?

    (a) Total parenteral nutrition (TPN)

    (b) Peripheral parenteral nutrition (PPN)

    (c) Total nutrient admixture (TNA)

    (d) I.V. fat emulsions (IVFEs)

4. Which of the following PN formulas is *most likely* to incite an allergic reaction during infusion?

    (a) Total parenteral nutrition (TPN)

    (b) Peripheral parenteral nutrition (PPN)

(c) Total nutrient admixture (TNA)

(d) I.V. fat emulsion (IVFE)

5. Which of the following methods of delivering PN is indicated most commonly for patients who are acutely ill?

   (a) Continuous

   (b) Cyclic

   (c) Peripheral

   (d) Gastric

6. All but which of the following medications may be admixed safely to either TPN or TNA solutions?

   (a) Insulin

   (b) Ondansetron (Zofran)

   (c) Famotidine (Pepcid)

   (d) Ranitidine (Zantac)

7. The most common complication associated with PN infusions is

   (a) sepsis.

   (b) bacteremia.

   (c) hyperglycemia.

   (d) hypoglycemia.

8. A systemic response that occurs when nutrients and fluids are administered too rapidly to a patient who is severely malnourished, causing heart failure, edema, and renal failure, is known as

   (a) hyperosmolar hyperglycemic nonketotic (HHNK) coma.

   (b) hepatic steatosis.

   (c) neurotoxic parkinsonism.

   (d) refeeding syndrome.

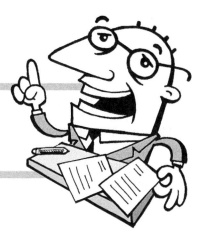

CHAPTER 11

Intravenous Pharmacologic Therapy

Learning Objectives

After completing this chapter, the learner will

1. Identify indications for intravenous (I.V.) pharmacologic therapy.

2. Describe basic guidelines for administration of I.V. pharmacologic agents.

3. Compare and contrast methods for delivering I.V. pharmacologic agents.

4. Identify adverse events that may occur from administration of I.V. pharmacologic agents and their prevention and treatment.

5. Recognize prototype drugs from classes of drugs that are commonly delivered by the I.V. route.

Key Terms

Pharmacologic agent	Attenuated
Compatible	Inactivated
Extravasation	Prototype drugs
Potentiated	

Indications for Intravenous (I.V.) Pharmacologic Therapy

The term *pharmacology* is rooted in the Greek word *pharmacon,* which translates to "drug" in English. Thus pharmacology refers to the study of medications or drugs, and a **pharmacologic agent** is another term for a medication or a drug. There are multiple indications for administering medications intravenously. These indications may include any or all of the following:

- The patient cannot swallow medications orally or absorb them enterally.

- Quicker drug action is required than can be accomplished by other routes.

- The medication has a very short half-life and must be administered continuously.

- A required medication is only effective when administered intravenously.

Almost any medication delivered by the I.V. route is more likely to cause venous access-site irritation and therefore is more likely to cause access-site thrombosis and phlebitis. Therefore, patients who receive I.V. medications should have those I.V. access sites scrutinized more carefully for these complications (see Chapter 6 for descriptions of thrombosis and phlebitis and their respective treatments).

SPEED BUMP

Medications delivered by the I.V. route are more likely to cause venous access-site irritation and therefore are more likely to cause access-site _____ and _____.

Basic Principles of Administering I.V. Pharmacologic Agents

There are some basic guidelines that must be followed whenever any medication is administered intravenously. These include the following:

- Only medications that are specifically manufactured and approved by the Food and Drug Administration (FDA) for I.V. use should be given intravenously.

- Medications should never be used past their expiration date because they can become unstable and less effective. Likewise, multiple-dose medication vials must be marked with the date on which they were opened and eventually discarded based on manufacturer's guidelines. Many medications expire 30 days after a vial is opened. Opened vials that are not dated should be discarded.

- Sterility of the medication and I.V. delivery system must be maintained during administration to prevent sepsis. The more often that the I.V. infusion setup is accessed, manipulated, or disrupted to administer medications, the greater is the likelihood that contamination will occur.

- Intravenous medications can be administered only with solutions verified as compatible. **Compatible** solutions and medications can be admixed without changing their potency or effectiveness. Mixing medications that are incompatible can result in inactivation of the medications, changed efficacy of the medications, or precipitation of crystals in the solution, which can become emboli when administered intravenously. By the same token, I.V. medications can be administered only in the same I.V. line with other I.V. medications after these medications are verified as compatible. If a single I.V. line is used to administer two medications that are incompatible, the line must be flushed with sufficient volume of solution compatible with both medications between administrations. Many medications are compatible with either 5% dextrose in water (D_5W) or 0.9% saline (i.e., normal saline [NS]) solutions.

- Manufacturer's guidelines must be followed whenever a medication is reconstituted or diluted with a solution (i.e., diluent). A medication that is reconstituted or diluted should be gently shaken to ensure that the medication is uniformly mixed with the solution. Likewise, medications admixed in I.V. bottles or bags should be gently shaken before administration.

- Medications that require reconstitution should be withdrawn from their vials with a filtered needle to prevent inclusion of any particles that could become blood-borne emboli if administered intravenously.

- Intravenous medications should be administered with needleless delivery devices to prevent needlestick injuries. Figure 11-1 shows commonly used needleless dispensing pins.

- Any medications that are admixed to any I.V. bag should be clearly labeled. The label should include the name of the medication, the medication dose, the initials of the person who prepared the medication, the date and time the medication was prepared, and the expiration date. The patient's name and another identifier such as the patient's hospital identification number also should be affixed to the I.V. bag on the label. The patient's room number is not considered a valid identifier.[6]

- The I.V. venous access site must be verified as patent prior to administering any medication.

- No matter what method of delivery is used, safety principles that guide the delivery of all medications must be followed. That is, the right patient should receive the right dose of the right medication by the right route at the right time. Dosages and time intervals for delivery of any I.V. medications must strictly adhere to pharmacy guidelines.

SPEED BUMP

Intravenous medications can be administered only with solutions verified as _____ .

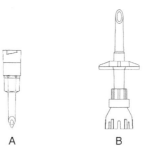

A   B

Figure 11-1   Needleless dispensing pins. *A.* Nonvented single-use pin. *B.* Nonvented multiple-use pin with two-way valve. (Courtesy of B. Braun, Products Catalog, 2005.)

Methods for Delivering I.V. Pharmacologic Agents 3

PERIPHERAL AND CENTRAL LINES

In many cases, it does not matter whether a medication is delivered into a peripheral line or a central line as long as the line is patent and there are no intraline solution or medication incompatibilities. Medications that should be delivered via a central line, if possible, are any medications that are vesicants. Vesicants can cause blistering of the vein. The likelihood of this occurring is lessened if the vesicant medication is diluted by coming into contact with more blood flow while it is infused. Central veins are larger vessels with greater flow than smaller vessels. Therefore, **extravasation**, which is the term used to define leaking of vesicant medication into tissues because of infiltration, is less likely to occur whenever a central line is used. Medications that are vesicants include many vasopressors (e.g., dobutamine [Dobutrex]).

CONTINUOUS DRIP INFUSION

Continuous drip medications typically are admixed to large-volume I.V. bags (e.g., 250, 500, and 1000 mL) and infused at a set hourly rate for several hours, days, or even indefinitely. In these instances, the I.V. administration setup can be either a primary or a secondary infusion set (e.g., piggybacked onto another primary infusion set) and may be delivered into a peripheral or central I.V. access site. The I.V. administration setup that delivers the medication should be attached to an electronic infusion device, such as a positive-pressure pump, otherwise called an *I.V. pump*. Figure 11-2 shows an example of a positive-pressure I.V. pump. These pumps and primary and secondary infusion sets are described in Chapter 3. Intravenous pumps reliably ensure that the medication is delivered at its intended hourly dosage.

Medications are delivered by continuous I.V. drip when they must be highly diluted in solution or when they have a very short half-life and must be delivered in small doses within short time intervals in order for the medication to maintain steady state and therapeutic effectiveness.[49] Examples of I.V. medications that are delivered continuously include adrenergic vasopressor agents such as dopamine (Dobutrex) and vasoconstrictor agents such as nitroprusside (Nipride).

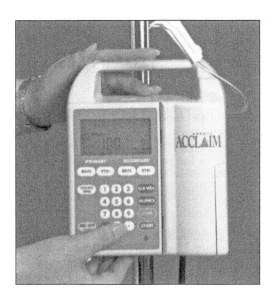

Figure 11-2 Positive-pressure infusion pump that features the ability to infuse piggybacked secondary medications. (Courtesy of Smith SF, Duell DJ, Martin BC: *Clinical Nursing Skills: Basic to Advanced Skills*, 7th ed. Upper Saddle River, NJ: Prentice-Hall, 2008:1092.)

CYCLIC INFUSION

Medications that are typically admixed to smaller I.V. bags (e.g., 50, 100, and 250 mL) and delivered to the I.V. access site at preset intervals are considered cyclic or intermittent I.V. infusions. In this case, the I.V. bags that contain the medication may be attached to a secondary infusion set and piggybacked onto the primary I.V. line, either infusing instead of the primary I.V. solution or infusing concomitant with the primary I.V. solution. Sometimes cyclic or intermittent I.V. medication bags can be set up to infuse into saline locks or other I.V. access ports and are flushed with saline or heparin solution after the infusion is complete.

Intravenous medications that tend to be delivered cyclically include most anti-infective agents, including antibiotics such as cefazolin (Ancef), antifungals such as amphotericin B (Fungizone), and antivirals such as acyclovir (Zovirax). No matter what method of delivery is used, the I.V. bags that contain medication (sometimes called I.V. piggyback, or IVPB bags) should be attached to an I.V. pump to ensure accurate delivery of the medication over the prescribed time interval. The I.V. pump can be programmed to ensure that the patient receives the dose of IVPB medication over the recommended time frame. For instance, suppose that a patient was prescribed to receive the following IVPB medication:

- 1 g cefazolin (Ancef) IVPB q8h

The pharmacy then prepares an IVPB bag with the following:

- 1 g cefazolin (Ancef) in 100 mL D_5W (i.e., 5% dextrose in water) to infuse over 30 minutes

Then the I.V. pump should be programmed to deliver the following:

- 100 mL solution at a rate of 200 mL/h

BOLUS/PUSH INFUSION

Delivery of a medication diluted with a small volume of solution and injected with a syringe directly into a port on an I.V. infusion set or a saline lock or other I.V. access port is referred to as a *bolus dose* or *I.V. push dose* of medication. Medications delivered by I.V. push are commonly ordered as one-time doses or on an "as needed" (i.e., PRN) basis.

Intravenous push medications may be prepared by the manufacturer or by a pharmacist in ready-to-administer syringes. However, it is not uncommon that the nurse is responsible for preparing the medication for I.V. push administration. It is essential that the nurse follows pharmacy guidelines that specify the volume of the diluent used to dilute the medication and that specifies the delivery rate. The nurse may need a watch with a second hand to time the approximate delivery time of the I.V. push medication. For instance, a medication that is commonly administered I.V. push in the acute-care setting is the loop diuretic furosemide (Lasix), and its recommended administration rate is no more than 20 mg/min.

If an I.V. push medication is administered into an I.V. line that is set up for continuous flow, the medication compatibility with the I.V. line solution must be verified prior to administration. Likewise, if any medications are admixed to the primary infusion setup or piggybacked into the primary infusion setup, their compatibility with the I.V. push medication must be verified. If the I.V. push medication is incompatible with the solution or any medications being delivered concomitantly with the I.V. administration setup, the line may be flushed with saline prior to and after administration of the I.V. push medication. If the I.V. push medication is administered into a saline lock or I.V. access port, these access sites also must be flushed with saline after delivery of the I.V. push medication and between dosages of medications.

PATIENT-CONTROLLED INFUSION

Patients may be able to self-administer their I.V. medications in the home setting (see Chapter 14). In addition to this, patients may be able to self-titrate dosages of analgesic agents to themselves in the acute-care setting on an as-needed basis using patient-controlled analgesia (PCA) pumps. PCA pumps typically are designed so that they use prefilled syringes of analgesic agents such as opioids (e.g., morphine sulfate). They can be programmed so that the patient receives a *basal rate* of the analgesic agent, which refers to a certain minimum hourly amount of analgesic solution that the PCA administers, and a *demand rate,* which is an "as needed" (i.e., PRN) dose that the patient may receive within a given time limit by pushing a button on the pump. These devices have a lock-out safety feature, and the dose may be changed only after a key is inserted into the setup. Figure 11-3 shows a PCA pump.

Any patient who is to use a PCA pump must be cognitively and physically capable of self-administering the analgesic agent. The patient's record should contain documentation that assessments were done to confirm this. Baseline pain assessments also should be done, along with periodic pain reassessments to evaluate responses to therapy. Prior to initiation of the analgesic therapy, the PCA pump and syringe should be validated by two health care professionals as containing the right medication that will be delivered in the right dosage by the right route at the right time to the right patient. Every time the analgesic syringe is changed, this validation must be repeated.[6]

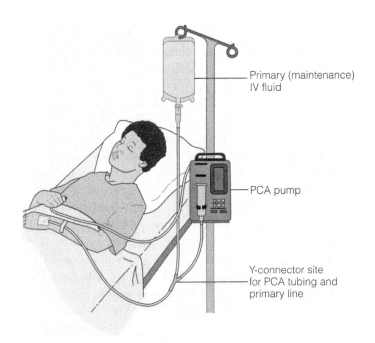

Primary (maintenance) IV fluid

PCA pump

Y-connector site for PCA tubing and primary line

Figure 11-3 Patient-controlled analgesia (PCA) pump. (Courtesy of Berman A, Snyder SJ, Kozier B, Erb GL: *Kozier & Erb's Fundamental's of Nursing,* 8th ed. Upper Saddle River, NJ: Prentice-Hall, 2008:121.)

Adverse Events

ALLERGIC AND ANAPHYLACTIC REACTIONS

Allergic and anaphylactic reactions can occur because the patient's immune system becomes primed to recognize the pharmacologic agent as foreign and forms immunoglobulin E (IgE) to attack what is perceived to be a foreign antigen. The immune response that is mounted in response to the administration of a medication may be mild or severe and life-threatening. Manifestations of mild allergic reactions include

- Flushing
- Urticaria (i.e., hives)
- Itching, particularly of the palms of the hands and soles of the feet

Allergic reactions may be delayed, and clinical signs and symptoms may not be exhibited until after the medication has infused. Whenever an allergic reaction to a medication is suspected, the physician should be notified, and the patient's clinical manifestations should be documented in the patient's record. If the medication is still infusing, it should be stopped immediately, prior to any other intervention. If another dose of the medication is slated to be administered, that dose should be held pending the physician's guidelines. The physician may order a dose of diphenhydramine (Benadryl), which may be administered orally or parenterally, to mitigate the allergic response.

An anaphylactic reaction is more severe than an allergic reaction and can progress to anaphylactic shock and cardiovascular collapse if untreated. In general, the quicker the onset of symptoms, the worse is the magnitude of the allergic or anaphylactic response. Manifestations of anaphylaxis include the same signs and symptoms as those of an allergic reaction with addition of the following:

- Wheezing with respiratory distress followed by stridor and laryngospasms
- Nausea, abdominal pains, severe cramping
- Tachycardia
- Hypotension with narrowed pulse pressure

Whenever anaphylaxis is suspected, the I.V. infusion of medication must be stopped immediately. The physician must be notified immediately. However, the I.V. line must be kept patent so that emergency medications can be infused.

These emergency medications may include epinephrine, diphenhydramine (Benadryl), and hydrocortisone (Solu-Cortef). Advanced cardiac life support (ACLS) guidelines may need to be followed as necessary.

EFFECTS OF INCOMPATIBILITY

Whenever an I.V. medication is infused, the solution that it is mixed with may not be compatible with the medication. In addition, the I.V. line that is chosen to administer the medication may infuse a second medication that is incompatible with the first medication. In these instances, incompatibility may cause several different adverse events. The effects of the medication may be stronger (i.e., **potentiated**), the effects of the medication may be weaker (i.e., **attenuated**), or the effects of the medication may be nil (i.e., **inactivated**). In some instances, mixing a medication with an incompatible solution or with another incompatible medication may cause a chemical reaction that results in the development of precipitate in the solution. When this precipitate is administered intravenously, it can cause venous irritation (i.e., phlebitis) and emboli (see Chapter 6 for a further discussion of phlebitis and emboli formation and their respective treatments).

Classes of I.V. Pharmacologic Agents, Methods of Delivery, and Incompatibilities

5 There are a multitude of medications that may be administered intravenously. It is not possible for any clinician to memorize each and every possible I.V. medication that might be prescribed for any given patient, its recommended method of I.V. delivery, and its attendant solution and medication incompatibilities. However, it is possible to identify general classes of drugs and the I.V. administration guidelines for prototype drugs in each of these classes. **Prototype drugs** are drugs that belong to a certain class of drugs and have effects that are representative of the other drugs in the class. Frequently, prototype drugs are the first drug marketed in a given drug class, but not always. Table 11-1 lists common classes of drugs that are administered intravenously, their respective prototype drugs, their recommended methods for I.V. administration, and their solution and drug incompatibilities.

Table 11-1 Classes of Common I.V. Pharmacologic Agents, Methods of Delivery, and Incompatibilities

Class	Prototype	Administration Guidelines*	Incompatibilities†
Antihistamines			
H$_1$-receptor antagonist	Diphenhydramine HCl (Benadryl)	IVP‡ May administer undiluted; administer 25 mg/min	Furosemide
Anti-infectives			
Antibiotics Aminoglycoside	Gentamicin sulfate (Garamycin)	Cyclic: Mix with 50–200 mL of D$_5$W or NS; infuse over 30 min–2 h	Fat emulsions Total parenteral nutrition Amphotericin B Ampicillin Azithromycin Cephalosporin Furosemide Heparin
β-Lactam	Imipenem-cilastatin (Primaxin)	Cyclic: Mix with 100 mL D$_5$W or NS; infuse over 20–30 min for each 500 mg medication infused	Lactated Ringer's Azithromycin
Cephalosporins First generation	Cefazolin sodium (Ancef)	Cyclic: Mix with 100 mL D$_5$W or NS; infuse over 5 min for each gram of medication infused	Aminoglycosides Cimetidine
Second generation	Cefoxitin (Mefoxin)	Cyclic: Mix with 50–100 mL D$_5$W or NS; infuse over 15 min	Aminoglycosides
Third generation	Cefotaxime sodium (Claforan)	Cyclic: Mix with 50–100 mL D$_5$W, NS, LR, or D$_5$½NS; infuse over 20–30 min	Aminoglycosides Sodium bicarbonate Vancomycin
Fourth generation	Cefepime (Maxipime)	Cyclic: Mix with 50–100 mL D$_5$W, NS, or D$_5$NS; infuse over 30 min	Aminoglycosides Metronidazole
Clindamycin	Clindamycin HCl (Cleocin)	Cyclic: Mix each 18 mg drug with a minimum of 1 mL D$_5$W, NS, or D$_5$½NS; infuse not to exceed 30 mg/min	Azithromycin Ciprofloxacin

(Continued)

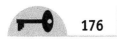

Table 11-1   (*Continued*)

Class	Prototype	Administration Guidelines*	Incompatibilities†
Macrolides Azalides	Azithromycin (Zithromax)	Cyclic: Mix with 250–500 mL D_5W, ½ NS, or D_5NS; infuse over at least 60 min	Cefotaxime Ciprofloxacin Furosemide Gentamycin Imipenem–cilastin Morphine
Penicillins Aminopenicillin	Ampicillin (Ampicen)	Cyclic: Mix with at least 50 mL NS, ½ NS, or LR; infuse over at least 15 min	Dextrose solutions
Antipseudomonal penicillin	Piperacillin	Cyclic: Mix with at least 50–100 mL D_5W or NS; infuse over 30 min	Aminoglycosides Amphotericin B
Extendedspec-trum penicillin	Ticarcillin (Ticar)	Cyclic: Mix with at least 50–100 mL D_5W or NS; infuse over 30–120 min	Aminoglycosides Amphotericin B Tetracyclines Vancomycin
Natural penicillin	Penicillin G potassium	Cyclic: Mix with at least 100 mL D_5W or NS; infuse over at least 60 min	Dextran Fat emulsions Amphotericin B Chlorpromazine Dopamine Metoclopramide Sodium bicarbonate Tetracyclines
Quinolones	Ciprofloxacin HCl (Cipro)	Cyclic: Mix with 100–250 mL D_5W or NS; infuse over 60 min	Ampicillin Azithromycin Cefepime Clindamycin Furosemide Heparin Phenytoin Sodium bicarbonate

Table 11-1 (*Continued*)

Class	Prototype	Administration Guidelines*	Incompatibilities†
Tetracycline	Doxycycline (Vibramycin)	Cyclic: Mix with at least 100 mL D_5W, NS, LR, or D_5LR; infuse over at least 60 min	Barbiturates Penicillins
Vancomycin	Vancomycin (Vancocin)	Cyclic: Mix with at least 200 mL D_5W, NS, or LR; infuse over at least 60 min	Albumin Barbiturates Cefepime Cefotaxime Cefoxitin Heparin Omeprazole Sodium bicarbonate Ticarcillin
Antifungal	Amphotericin B (Fungizone)	Cyclic: Recommended preparation with solution; infusion time variable	Saline Total perenteral nutrition Any other drugs
Antiprotozoal	Metronidazole (Flagyl)	Cyclic: Most frequently supplied in premixed I.V. bagsbags that contain 5 mEq sodium bicarbonate/500 mg metronidazole; infuse over 60 min	Total parenteral nutrition Amphotericin B Dopamine
Antiviral	Acyclovir (Zovirax)	Cyclic: Mix with D_5W, NS, or LR to yield 5 mg/mL; infuse over 60 min	Bacteriostatic water Albumin Hespan Total parenteral nutrition Dopamine
Autonomic nervous system agents			
Adrenergic agonists α-Adrenergic agonist	Methoxamine HCl (Vasoxyl)	IVP: May administer undiluted; administer 5 mg/min Continuous: Mix 20 mg in 250 mL D_5W; titrate to maintain systolic BP > 60 mm Hg This drug is a vesicant; therefore, administer in a central I.V. line, if possible	Sodium bicarbonate

(*Continued*)

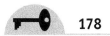

Table 11-1 *(Continued)*

Class	Prototype	Administration Guidelines*	Incompatibilities†
α- & β-Adrenergic agonist	Epinephrine	IVP: *Caution:* be certain to use 1:10,000 strength, which doses 0.1 mg epinephrine in 1 mL; an alternate strength of 1:1000 strength is available, which doses 1.0 mg epinephrine in 1 mL solution; this is most frequently administered during ACLS protocols and may be given as a quick, nontimed bolus dose Continuous: Mix 1:1000 strength in 250–500 mL D_5W; begin at 1 µg/min; titrate as indicated up to 10 µg/min	Ampicillin Sodium bicarbonate
β-Adrenergic agonist	Isoproterenol HCl (Isuprel)	IVP: Mix 1 mL of 1:5000 strength with 9 mL D_5W or NS to yield 1:50,000 strength, or 0.02 mg/mL; administer 0.02 mg/min Continuous: Mix 10 mL of 1:5000 strength in 500 mL D_5W; begin with bolus of 0.02–0.06 mg, followed by 5 µg/min infusion	Sodium bicarbonate
Selective $β_1$-adrenergic agonist	Dopamine (Dobutrex)	Continuous: Mix 200 mg in 250 or 500 mL of D_5W, NS, D_5NS, $D_5\frac{1}{2}NS$, or D_5LR to yield 800 or 400 µg/mL, respectively; begin infusion at 2 µg/kg/min; titrate up to 5 µg/kg/min for renal effects; begin infusion at 2–5 µg/kg/min; titrate up to 10 µg/kg/min for vasopressor effects This drug is a vesicant; therefore, administer in a central I.V. line, if possible.	Acyclovir Amphotericin B Ampicillin Penicillin G potassium Sodium bicarbonate

Table 11-1 *(Continued)*

Class	Prototype	Administration Guidelines*	Incompatibilities†
Adrenergic antagonists α-Antagonist	Labetalol (Normodyne)	IVP: May administer undiluted; administer 20 mg/2 min; Continuous: Mix in 250 mL D_5W, NS, LR, or D_5NS to yield 1 mg/mL solution; administer at 2 mg/min	Furosemide Heparin Sodium bicarbonate
β-Antagonist	Propranolol HCl (Inderal)	IVP: May administer undiluted; administer 1 mg/min Cyclic: Mix prescribed dose in 50 mL NS; infuse over 15–20 min	Amphotericin B
Cholinergics Cholinesterase inhibitor	Neostigmine (Prostigmin)	IVP: May administer undiluted; administer 0.5 mg/min	None of note
Benzodiazepine antagonist	Flumazenil (Mazicon)	IVP: May administer undiluted; administer 0.2 mg/15 s	None of note
Blood formers, coagulants, and anticoagulants			
Anticoagulants	Heparin sodium	Continuous: Mix with 5000–20,000 units heparin to 250–1000 mL D_5W, NS, or LR to desired concentration; infuse loading dose of hydrocortisone approximately 5000 units followed by maintenance dose based on kg weight and anticoagulation effectiveness noted on aPTT	Chlorpromazine Diazepam Doxycycline Gentamycin Hydrocortisone Morphine Nitroglycerin Phenytoin Vancomycin
Direct thrombin inhibitor	Lepirudin (Refludan)	IVP: Reconstitute as directed by manufacturer with D_5W, NS, or sterile water to yield 5 mg/mL; reconstituted solution remains stable for only 24 h; administer 0.4 mg/kg as bolus over 15–20 s Continuous: Mix 100 mg in 250–500 mL D_5W or NS; begin at 0.15 mg/kg/h; titrate to achieve anticoagulane effectiveness as noted on aPTT	None of note

(Continued)

Table 11-1   *(Continued)*

Class	Prototype	Administration Guidelines*	Incompatibilities†
Antiplatelet agents Glycoprotein IIb/ IIIa inhibitor	Abciximab	IVP: May administer undiluted; administer 0.5 mg/kg over 5 min as bolus dose Continuous: Mix 4.5 mL (9.0 mg) into 250 mL of D_5W or NS; infuse after bolus at a rate not to exceed 10 µg/min (i.e., 17 mL/h)	Any other drugs
Hematopoietic growth factor	Epoetin alfa (Procrit)	IVP: May administer undiluted; administer full dose over 1 min	Any other drugs
Hemostatic	Aminocaproic acid (Amicar)	Continuous: Dilute each gram with 50 mL D_5W, NS, or LR; infuse bolus of 5 g in 250 mL over first hour, followed by 1 g in 50 mL/h as indicated	None of note
Thrombolytic	Alteplase (Activase)	Reconstitute 50- or 100-mg single-use vials per manufacturer's instructions with nitroglycerin diluent supplied by manufacturer *For acute coronary syndrome:* IVP: Give 6–10% of total dose as bolus over 1–2 min Continuous: After IVP bolus is administered, infuse remainder of 60% total dose within first hour of treatment; divide remaining 40% of total dose; infuse over 2 h *For pulmonary embolism:* Continuous: Infuse dose over 2 h *For ischemic cerebrovascular accident:* IVP: Administer 5-mg bolus over 1 min Continuous: After bolus, infuse 0.75 mg/kg over 1 h	Dopamine Heparin Nitroglycerin Any other drugs

Table 11-1 *(Continued)*

Class	Prototype	Administration Guidelines*	Incompatibilities†
Cardiovascular agents			
Antiarrhythmic agents			
Class IA	Procainamide HCl (Pronestyl)	IVP: Mix 100 mg in 5–10 mL D$_5$W or sterile water; administer 20 mg/min Continuous: Mix 1 g in 250–500 mL D$_5$W to yield 4 or 2 mg/mL, respectively; infuse after bolus at 2–6 mg/min	Inamrinone
Class IB	Lidocaine HCl	IVP: May administer undiluted; administer 50 mg/min Continuous: Mix 1 g in 250–500 mL D$_5$W to yield 4 or 2 mg/mL, respectively; infuse after bolus at 1–4 mg/min	Amphotericin B Ampicillin Cefazolin Phenytoin
Class II	Propanolol HCl	See coverage in previous section under Autonomic Nervous System Agents: Adrenergic Antagonists: β-antagonist	
Class III	Amiodarone HCl	Continuous: Loading dose: Mix 150 mg with 100 mL D$_5$W; infuse this loading dose over 10 min Second infusion: Mix 960 mg with 500 mL D$_5$W; infuse 1 mg/min over first 6 hours; then drop rate to 0.5 mg/min over next 18 h Maintenance infusion: May mix same solution as for second infusion; infuse at 0.5 mg/min This drug is a vesicant; therefore, administer in a central I.V. line, if possible	Cefazolin Digoxin Heparin Imipenem–cilastin Magnesium sulfate Nitroprusside Piperacillin Sodium bicarbonate

(Continued)

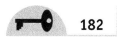

Table 11-1   (*Continued*)

Class	Prototype	Administration Guidelines*	Incompatibilities†
Calcium channel antagonists	Verapamil (Calan)	IVP: May administer undiluted; administer 5–10 mg over 2–3 min	Albumin Amphotericin B Ampicillin Hydralazine Sodium bicarbonate
Cardiac glycoside	Digoxin (Lanoxin)	IVP: May administer undiluted; administer each dose over at least 5 min	Amiodarone
Central-acting antihypertensive	Methyldopa (Aldomet)	Cyclic: Mix in 100–200 mL D_5W to yield 10 mg/mL; infuse over 30–60 min	Fat emulsions Amphotericin B Verapamil
Inotropic agent	Inamrinone lactate (Inocor)	IVP: May administer undiluted; administer loading dose over 2–3 min Continuous: Mix 300 mg in 60 mL solution with an additional 60 mL NS or ½ NS to yield 2.5 mg/mL; infuse after loading dose is administered at rate of 2.5–10.0 µg/kg/min	Dextrose solutions Furosemide Sodium bicarbonate
Nitrate vasodilator	Nitroglycerin (Nitrostat)	Continuous: May administer in premixed bottles; may mix to variable concentration, of 25–500 µg/mL; infuse with starting dose of 5 µg/min; titrate to effectiveness	Use only glass bottles and special tubing as drug becomes unstable when in contact with plastic Alteplase Hydralazine Phenytoin
Nonnitrate vasodilator	Hydralazine HCl (Apresoline)	IVP: May administer undiluted; administer 10 mg/min	Ampicillin Hydrocortisone Nitroglycerin Phenobarbital Verapamil

Table 11-1   (*Continued*)

Class	Prototype	Administration Guidelines*	Incompatibilities†
Central nervous system agents			
Analgesics			
Opioids	Morphine sulfate	IVP: Mix 2–10 mg in at least 5 mL sterile water; administer single doses over 4–5 min	Amphotericin B Azithromycin Cefepime Heparin Phenobarbital Phenytoin Sodium bicarbonate
Opioid agonist-santagonists	Pentazocine HCl (Talwin)	IVP: May administer undiluted; administer 5 mg/min	Barbiturates Heparin Sodium bicarbonate
Opioid antagonist	Naloxone HCl (Narcan)	IVP: May administer undiluted; administer 0.4 mg/10–15 seconds	Amphotericin B
Anticonvulsants			
Barbiturate	Phenobarbital (Luminal)	IVP: Mix dose with 10 mL sterile water; administer 60 mg/min	Albumin Total parenteral nutrition Amphotericin B Chlorpromazine Hydralazine Hydrocortisone Insulin Morphine Tetracyclines Vancomycin
Central Nervous system depressant	Magnesium sulfate	IVP: May give undiluted if concentration is ≤ 20%; administer 150 mg/min Continuous: Mix 4 G in 250 mL D_5W; infuse over 4 h	Fat emulsions Amiodarone Amphotericin B Cefepime Sodium bicarbonate
Gamma amino butyric acid (GABA) inhibitor	Valproic acid sodium (Valproate)	Cyclic: Mix dose in at least 50 mL D_5W, NS, or LR; administer over at least 60 min	None of note

(*Continued*)

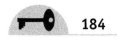
Table 11-1 *(Continued)*

Class	Prototype	Administration Guidelines*	Incompatibilities†
Hydantoin	Phenytoin (Dilantin)	IVP: May administer undiluted; administer 25–50 mg/min	Dextrose solutions Total parenteral nutrition Amphotericin B Ciprofloxacin Clindamycin Insulin Lidocaine Morphine Nitroglycerin Potassium chloride
Anxiolytics Benzodiazepine	Diazepam (Valium)	IVP: May administer undiluted; administer 5 mg/min	Furosemide Heparin Morphine Potassium chloride
Antipsychotics Phenothiazine	Chlorpromazine (Thorazine)	IVP: Mix 25 mg with 24 mL NS to yield 1 mg/mL; administer 1 mg/min Continuous: Mix 25 mg with a maximum of 1000 mL NS; infuse at a maximum dose of 1 mg/min	Aminophylline B Ampicillin Cefepime Cimetidine Furosemide Heparin Penicillin G Phenobarbital
Electrolyte and fluid balance agents			
Acidifying agent	Ammonium chloride	Cyclic: Mix 20-mL vial in 500 mL NS; infuse at no more than 5 mL/min	Sodium bicarbonate

Table 11-1   (*Continued*)

Class	Prototype	Administration Guidelines*	Incompatibilities†
Alkalinizing agent	Sodium bicarbonate	IVP: May administer undiluted; administer IVP per ACLS protocols in nontimed bolus Continuous: May mix 50 mEq/50 mL in 1000 mL D_5W, NS, $D_5\frac{1}{2}NS$, or D_5NS; infuse no more than 50 mEq/h over no more than 8 h before patient's acid–base status is reevaluated	Fat emulsions Lactated Ringer's (LR) Ammonium hydrochloride Calcium gluconate Cefotaxime Chlorpromazine Dopamine Imipenem–cilastin Insulin Isoproterenol Labetalol Magnesium sulfate Metoclopramide Morphine Penicillin G potassium Pentazocine Phenobarbital Vancomycin
Diuretics Loop	Furosemide (Lasix)	IVP: May administer undiluted; administer at 20 mg/min	Total parenteral nutrition Azithromycin Chlorpromazine Ciprofloxacin Diazepam Diphenhydramine Dopamine Gentamicin Hydralazine Isoproterenol Labetalol Metoclopramide Morphine Ondansetron Prochlorperazine
Osmotic	Mannitol (Osmitrol)	IVP: May administer undiluted; administer over 30–90 min	Cefepime Imipenem–cilastin Potassium chloride

(*Continued*)

Table 11-1   (*Continued*)

Class	Prototype	Administration Guidelines*	Incompatibilities†
Replacement solutions			
Calcium	Calcium gluconate	IVP: May administer undiluted; administer 10% strength at 0.5 mL/min Continuous: Mix 10% dose in 1000 mL NS; infuse at rate not to exceed 200 mg/min This drug is a vesicant; therefore, administer in a central I.V. line, if possible	Amphotericin B Metoclopramide
Potassium	Potassium chloride	*Caution:* Do *not* administer IVP Continuous: Mix in concentration not to exceed 80 mEq/L for administration through central I.V. lines, and in concentrations not to exceed 40 mEq/L for administration through peripheral I.V. lines; infuse at rate not to exceed 10 mEq/h	Amphotericin B Diazepam Phenytoin
Gastrointestinal agents			
Antiemetics	Prochlorperazine (Compazine)	IVP: Mix 5 mg in 1 mL solution with 4 mL NS; administer 5 mg/min Cyclic: Mix 5–10 mg with 50–100 mL D_5W or NS; infuse over 15–30 min	Amphotericin B Ampicillin Calcium gluconate Cefepime Furosemide Hydrocortisone Morphine Phenobarbital Sodium bicarbonate

Table 11-1 (*Continued*)

Class	Prototype	Administration Guidelines*	Incompatibilities†
5-HT$_3$ antagonist	Ondansetron HCl (Zofran)	IVP: May administer undiluted; administer dose over at least 30 s Cyclic: May mix with 50 mL D$_5$W or NS and infuse over 15 min	Total parenteral nutrition Acyclovir Amphotericin B Ampicillin Cefepime Furosemide Piperacillin
Antisecretory	Cimetidine (Tagamet)	IVP: Mix 300 mg in 18 mL D$_5$W or NS; administer over at least 5 min Cyclic: Mix 300 mg in 50 mL D$_5$W or NS; infuse over 15–20 min Continuous: Mix 300 mg in 1000 mL crystalloid solution; infuse over 24 h	Amphotericin B Cefazolin Cefepime Chlorpromazine
Prokinetic	Metoclopramide HCl (Reglan)	IVP: May administer undiluted dosages ≤10 mg; administer over 1–2 min Cyclic: Mix with 50 mL D$_5$W or NS; infuse over 15 min	Amphotericin B Ampicillin Calcium gluconate Cefepime Furosemide Penicillin G potassium Sodium bicarbonate Tetracyclines
Hormones			
Antidiabetic	Insulin, regular	IVP: May administer undiluted; administer 50 units/min Continuous: Mix 10 units in 100 mL NS; infusion rate variable	Phenobarbital Phenytoin Sodium bicarbonate
Antidiuretic	Vasopressin (Pitressin)	Continuous: May mix with D$_5$W or NS to yield 0.1–1.0 units/mL; infusion rate variable	None of note

(*Continued*)

Table 11-1   (*Continued*)

Class	Prototype	Administration Guidelines*	Incompatibilities†
Corticosteroids	Hydrocortisone sodium succinate (Solu-cortef)	IVP: May administer undiluted; administer dose over 1 min Cyclic: May mix dose with 50–100 mL D_5W or NS; infuse over 10 min	Ampicillin Chlorpromazine Ciprofloxacin Diazepam Diphenhydramine Furosemide Heparin Hydralazine Lidocaine Magnesium sulfate Phenobarbital Phenytoin Prochlorperazine Vancomycin
Oxytocic	Oxytocin (Pitocin)	Continuous: Mix 10 units in 1000 mL D_5W or NS *To induce labor:* Begin infusion at 1 mU/min; titrate as needed *For postpartum bleeding:* Infuse at 20–40 mU/min	Prochlorperazine

*Dosage guidelines generally pertain to adults.

†This list of incompatibilities is noninclusive. It contains only common solutions and incompatibilities with other prototype drugs listed on this table.

‡IVP refers to intravenous push

Summary

The same principles that guide safe and effective administration of all medications guide administration of I.V. medications. That is, the right patient must receive the right dose of the right medication by the right route at the right time. The nurse must be cognizant of basic principles that guide effective and safe delivery of I.V. medications and must be competent in operating a variety of I.V. delivery systems to administer I.V. medications effectively.

Quiz

1. Which of the following is an indication for administering a medication by the I.V. route?

   (a) A patient would prefer to not swallow a medication

   (b) Quick drug action can be ensured only by administering the medication intravenously

   (c) The medication to be delivered has a long half-life

   (d) The required medication is effective when it is given intravenously

2. Which of the following is *not* a guiding principle for administration of I.V. pharmacologic agents?

   (a) Only medications approved by the FDA for I.V. use should be given intravenously

   (b) Medications maintain their stability long after their expiration date and still may be given intravenously

   (c) Medications that must be reconstituted should be withdrawn from their vials with a filtered needle

   (d) Intravenous medications should be administered with needleless delivery devices

3. All but which of the following must be included on I.V. bags with admixed medications?

   (a) The patient's name

   (b) The patient's room number

   (c) The name of the medication

   (d) The dose of the medication

4. Intravenous medications that should be delivered via a central line if at all possible are those that cause

   (a) extravasation.

   (b) potentiation.

   (c) attenuation.

   (d) inactivation.

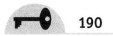

5. A patient is slated to receive a dose of an IVPB antibiotic over 60 minutes. The medication is admixed to a 100-mL bag. The I.V. pump is correctly set to infuse 100 mL of solution at what rate of infusion?

(a) 50 mL/h

(b) 100 mL/h

(c) 150 mL/h

(d) 200 mL/h

6. Which of the following patients is eligible to use a PCA pump?

(a) An infant who is postoperative for repair of a cleft palate

(b) A 40-year-old patient with quadriplegia who is postoperative for debridement of a pressure ulcer

(c) An 80-year-old patient with advanced dementia who is hospitalized for severe sepsis

(d) A cognitively intact and otherwise healthy 30-year-old man who is postoperative after donating a kidney to his brother

7. The nurse begins to administer an IVPB dose of penicillin G when the patient suddenly complains of dyspnea and itching of the palms of the hands. The nurse's best first action is to

(a) stop the infusion.

(b) call the physician.

(c) disconnect the I.V. administration setup and venous access.

(d) verify the patient's allergies.

8. When a medication is administered intravenously with an incompatible solution and its effects then becomes stronger, its pharmacologic effects are said to be

(a) extravasated.

(b) potentiated.

(c) attenuated.

(d) inactivated.

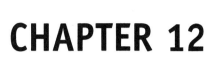

CHAPTER 12

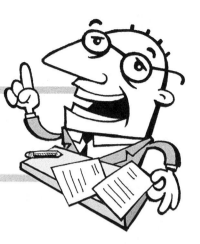

Intravenous Therapy and Infants and Children

Learning Objectives

After completing this chapter, the learner will

1   Identify developmental stages in infants and children.

2   Describe differences in intravenous (I.V.) delivery systems and I.V. access devices that are indicated for use in infants and children from those indicated for use in adults.

3   Recognize basic competencies that must be mastered by nurses who administer I.V. therapy to infants and children.

4 Identify alternate infusion access sites that might be used in infants and children.

5 Discuss guidelines for administration of I.V. crystalloids, blood components, parenteral nutrients, and medications in infants and children.

 Key Terms

Infancy	School-aged
Toddler	Adolescence
Preschool	Intraosseous

Indications for Intravenous (I.V.) Therapy in Infants and Children

The indications for I.V. therapy in infants and children are the same as the indications for I.V. therapy in adults. That is, I.V. therapy is indicated to achieve or maintain fluid and electrolyte balance, replace or supplement needed blood components, provide nutrients, and administer medications. Among children, some of the most common reasons to initiate I.V. therapy are to correct dehydration that occurs most commonly from gastroenteritis and to administer I.V. antibiotics.[50,51]

1 Specific guidelines for treating infants and children vary considerably based on developmental stage. These developmental stages include the following:

- **Infancy:** birth to 12 months and 3–6 kg weight
- **Toddler:** 1–2 years and 6–12 kg weight
- **Preschool:** 4–6 years and 12–15 kg weight
- **School-aged:** 6–12 years and 16–35 kg weight
- **Adolescence:** 13–19 years and >35 kg weight

Whenever relevant, differences in treatment of infants and children based on developmental stage will be addressed throughout this chapter. This chapter will provide a cursory overview of some of the basic principles for administering I.V. therapy in infants and children. The reader is encouraged to review additional sources of information to find more specific and comprehensive content on I.V. therapy and infants and children.

Selecting I.V. Therapy Delivery Systems for Infants and Children

INFUSION SETS

2 Intravenous line sets that are used in infants and children are similar to those used in adults. Adolescents who are similar in size to adults (e.g., ≥45 kg) typically use the same types of I.V. line sets that are used in adults. Infants, younger children, and smaller-sized adolescents cannot tolerate the larger volumes of fluids, blood components, nutrients, and medications that are indicated in adults, and the I.V. administration sets therefore must be capable of delivering lesser amounts of solution. Sometimes, smaller I.V. containers (i.e., I.V. bottles and bags) are hung. In most instances, either the primary infusion set uses a minidrop drip chamber, or the I.V. bag drips into a volume-limited chamber that also has a minidrop drip chamber.

Most minidrop infusion sets, sometimes called *pediatric infusion sets,* deliver 50–60 drops/mL of solution rather than the conventional or macrodrop primary infusion sets that deliver 10–20 drops/mL of solution. Minidrop infusion sets can be distinguished visually from macrodrop infusion sets because there is a drip needle in the center of the drip chamber of the minidrop set that delivers smaller drops than can be delivered with a macrodrip chamber. Figure 12-1 shows a commonly used microdrop infusion set.

SPEED BUMP

Minidrop infusion sets can be distinguished visually from macrodrop infusion sets because there is a drip needle in the center of the drip chamber of the minidrop set that delivers _____ than can be delivered with a macrodrip chamber.

Volume-limited chambers also can be used to ensure delivery of small quantities of fluid. These are designed with a typical spike to access the I.V. bag. The desired amount of fluid then is infused into the volume chamber, also referred to as the *burette chamber,* which then is titrated at the desired rate by a microdrop drip chamber. Most volume chambers are limited in size to contain no more than 150 mL of fluid. There are access ports on these volume chambers that can be used to add medications that might need to be diluted with solution and infused on a cyclic basis, including most I.V. antibiotics. Figure 12-2 shows a commonly used volume-limited chamber infusion set.

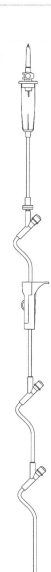

Figure 12-1 Primary minidrop I.V. administration setup. (Courtesy of B. Braun, Products Catalog, 2005.)

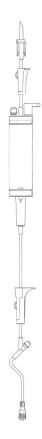

Figure 12-2   Primary minidrop I.V. administration setup with 150-mL burette chamber. (Courtesy of B. Braun, Products Catalog, 2005.)

ELECTRONIC INFUSION DEVICES

Most infants and children should receive I.V. therapy by electronic infusion devices, otherwise called *I.V. pumps.* Many brands of I.V. pumps used for adults also can be used to deliver I.V. fluids to infants and children because they can be programmed to deliver small volumes of fluid reliably and accurately. However, when infants and children require the delivery of very small dosages of fluids, including I.V. medications, these small dosages may be delivered most reliably and accurately by a pump that exerts positive pressure on a syringe rather than an I.V. bag. These types of special electronic infusion devices are called *syringe pumps.* Many syringe pumps can accommodate syringes that range in size from 1–30 mL.[52] Figure 12-3 shows a commonly used syringe pump.

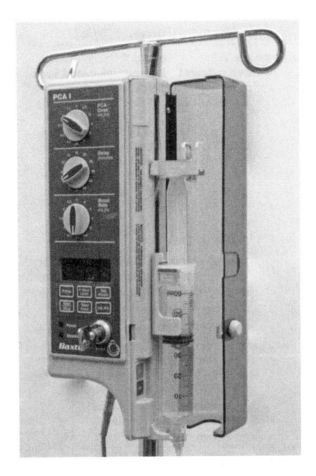

Figure 12-3   Syringe pump. (From Berman A, Snyder SJ, Kozier B. Courtesy Erb GL. *Fundamentals of Nursing,* 8th ed. Upper Saddle River, NJ: Prentice-Hall, 2008, p 881.)

Patient Preparation

Prior to initiating I.V. therapy, the nurse must verify that an appropriate prescriptive order has been written by a physician or other advanced-practice clinician recognized by the respective state board of nursing as having the authority to prescribe this type of interventional therapy. Authorized advanced-practice clinicians may include nurse practitioners, nurse midwives, nurse anesthetists, or physician assistants. In general, those preparatory guidelines outlined in Chapters 4 and 5 as appropriate for adult patients who are slated to begin I.V. therapy by either peripheral or central I.V. access routes are also appropriate for infants and children.[6]

Informed consent should be obtained from the infant's or the child's legal representative prior to initiating I.V. therapy. Whenever possible, assent also should be solicited from the school-aged child or adolescent who is scheduled to begin I.V. therapy.[6]

SPEED BUMP

Informed consent should be obtained from the infant's or child's legal representative prior to initiating I.V. therapy. Whenever possible, _____ also should be solicited from the school-aged child or adolescent who is scheduled to begin I.V. therapy.

---

3 The nurse who is responsible for initiating I.V. therapy in infants and children at a minimum must be

- Comfortable and competent in finding appropriate vascular access routes in infants and children

- Cognizant of the physiologic and psychological differences among infants and children who represent different developmental stages

- Comfortable and competent in working with I.V. therapy equipment tailor-made for infants and children[6]

Any child slated to have an I.V. access device inserted should have the procedure explained to him or her in words that are readily understandable. Some pediatrics experts advocate that preschool-aged and school-aged children feel less helpless when confronted by unpleasant procedures if they are permitted to see and touch the equipment in advance. Adolescents tend to respond better to procedures when they are permitted to make choices, so giving the adolescent the option to help select a reasonable I.V. access site might be a good coping strategy. For most children, it is comforting to know where their parents or caregivers are and when they can expect to see them again. Some pediatrics experts advocate letting parents and caregivers stay with children during I.V. initiation, believing that it reduces anxiety on the part of the children as well as the parents and caregivers.[53]

The *Infusion Nursing Standards of Practice* (2006) published by the Infusion Nurses Society advocates that "use of topical anesthetics prior to painful dermal procedures in children should be encouraged, in addition to use of adjunctive and less invasive anxiolytic therapies" (Standard 40, p. S41).[6] Topical anesthetics that might be applied to numb the pain from the needle used to gain vascular access include lidocaine and prilocaine creams (i.e., EMLA cream). The disadvantage to use of topical creams is that they must be applied for at least 1 hour before they are effective. This precludes their usefulness in infants and children who must have their I.V. therapy initiated emergently.

Peripheral I.V. Therapy

SELECTION OF VASCULAR ACCESS SITES

Selection of peripheral I.V. access sites in infants and children follows the same general guidelines noted in Chapter 4 for adults. The same veins that are preferred access sites in adults are preferred access sites in infants and children, and they are found in approximately the same anatomic locations. Gaining vascular access may be more difficult in the infant or child, however, because the veins are smaller and more fragile.

There are additional peripheral access sites that might be used in the infant and sometimes the toddler if the dorsal metacarpal, cephalic, basilic, median cephalic, and median cubital veins cannot be accessed. These veins include the scalp veins and the feet and ankle veins. When scalp veins are accessed, the tip of the needle should face downward, toward the infant's chest.[52] Although scalp veins are readily accessible in infants, their use is most disagreeable to parents, and they may be more prone to infiltration. Figure 12-4 shows commonly accessed scalp veins in an infant.

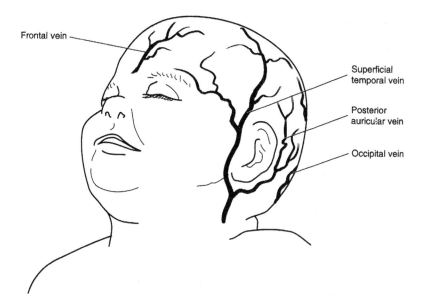

Figure 12-4   Infant scalp veins. (Used with permission from Hankins J, Lonsway RAW, Hedrick C, Perdue MB: *The Infusion Nurses Society: Infusion Therapy in Clinical Practice,* 2nd ed. Philadelphia: Saunders, 2001.)

Prior to selection of an I.V. access site, children should receive the same consideration that adults receive concerning arm dominance. It is important for children who have developed dominance to be able to continue to manipulate their world and to play. Play is therapeutic to children, and if an I.V. access site is selected on the dominant arm, the child's ability to play will be hampered.[50]

SELECTION OF VASCULAR ACCESS DEVICES

Vascular access devices used in adults also can be used in infants and children. Steel-winged infusion devices and short and midline over-the-needle catheters are indicated for the same use in infants and children as they are in adults. In general, the gauges used for children are smaller than those used for adults and can be as small as 24- or 26-G catheters or 25- and 27-G butterfly needles. These types of devices are described in greater detail in Chapter 4.

Central I.V. Therapy

SELECTION OF VASCULAR ACCESS SITES

Selection of central I.V. access sites in infants and children follows the same general guidelines noted in Chapter 5 for adults. The same veins that are preferred central access sites in adults are preferred central access sites in infants and children, and they are found in approximately the same anatomic locations. As is true with peripheral I.V. therapy, gaining vascular access may be more difficult in the infant or child, however, because the veins are smaller and more fragile. Additional central access sites that might be used in a child include the veins of the head and lower extremities,[6] including the femoral vein.

SELECTION OF VASCULAR ACCESS DEVICES

Vascular access devices that are appropriate for gaining central I.V. access in infants and children are similar to those used in adults but are smaller in size and length. The diameter of central I.V. access devices in infants and children might be referred to in gauge or sometimes in French sizes (e.g., 20 G is approximately the same as 3 French). Chapter 5 discusses the sizes and characteristics of a number of central vascular access devices. In general, peripherally inserted central catheters (PICCs)

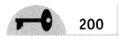

have become commonplace devices for safely and efficacy in infusing fluids, nutrients, and medications in children who require I.V. therapy for more than 7 days.[54,55] In addition, PICCs are useful devices for withdrawing blood specimens from children who require frequent monitoring of blood results without necessitating the trauma of repeated venipuncture.[56]

Alternative Infusion Therapy Delivery Sites 4

INTRAOSSEOUS

In emergency situations when it is not possible to gain either peripheral or central venous access expeditiously, the medullary cavity of the long bones, or the **intraosseous** site, may provide a reasonable alternative for delivery of crystalloids and blood components to infants, toddlers, and preschool children. The first-line site that should be accessed for this purpose is the anteromedial aspect of the tibia (Fig. 12-5). Alternate sites might include the distal medial tibia, midanterior distal femur, iliac crest, and humerus.[52] Bones with suspected fractures may not be accessed for this purpose. Access may be achieved with either specially designed intraosseous needles or generic straight needles that may vary in size from 16–19 G. Only clinicians specially trained in this technique may use this approach to fluid or blood component resuscitation. Patients should not receive fluids or blood components by this route for longer than 24 hours.[52]

UMBILICAL VEINS AND ARTERIES

Newborn infants who experience life-threatening conditions may be candidates for the insertion of either umbilical venous catheters (UVCs) or umbilical arterial catheters (UACs). Both these methods of vascular access should be performed only by neonatologists or neonatal nurse practitioners. Typically, neonates receiving this kind of I.V. therapy are in neonatal intensive-care units (NICUs). The nurse caring for neonates requiring this special type of therapy should receive special education in caring for neonates and training in competent delivery of this special type of I.V. therapy.

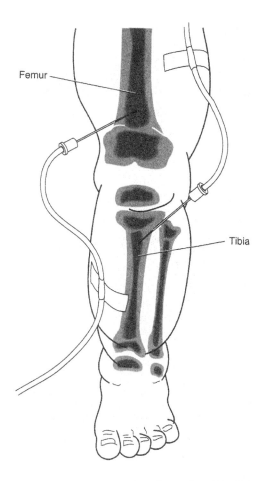

Figure 12-5 Pediatric intraosseus access site. (From Hankins J, Lonsway RAW, Hedrick C, Perdue MB: *The Infusion Nurses Society: Infusion Therapy in Clinical Practice,* 2nd ed. Philadelphia: Saunders, 2001.)

Delivery of I.V. Therapy in Infants and Children 5

CRYSTALLOIDS

Intravenous infusion of crystalloids might be indicated in infants and children who are dehydrated or who have a disruption in electrolyte balance. In general, infants and children have a lesser proportion of fluid that comprises their body mass than do adults. Therefore, infants and children are more sensitive to losses of fluid than are adults.

Infants and children who appear to be moderately or severely dehydrated may need an initial fluid bolus of 20 mL/kg of body weight of lactated Ringer's (LR) or 0.9% normal saline (NS), followed by a maintenance infusion of crystalloids calculated based on body weight. General rules for maintenance infusions following the fluid bolus include the following:

- If less than 10 kg body weight, then infuse 100 ml/kg over 24 hours.
- If 11–20 kg body weight, then infuse 1000 mL plus 50 mL/kg over 24 hours for each kilogram over 10 kg body weight.
- If 21–30 kg body weight, then infuse 1500 mL plus 20 mL/kg over 24 hours for each kilogram over 20 kg body weight.

The choice of the crystalloid for infusion depends on whether the child is suffering from isotonic, hypertonic, or hypotonic dehydration and the relative status of key serum electrolytes. Chapter 2 provides an overview of isotonic, hypertonic, and hypotonic states. After the maintenance infusion rate is calculated, dehydrated children's total fluid requirements then are further stratified based on whether they are mildly, moderately, or severely dehydrated. The final calculated fluid replacement needs for the next 24 hours is based on the following formula:

- If the child is mildly dehydrated, then fluid replacement needs include the calculated maintenance rate *plus* an additional one-half of the maintenance rate.
- If the child is moderately dehydrated, then the fluid replacement needs are *twice* the calculated maintenance rate.
- If the child is severely dehydrated, then the fluid replacement needs are *twice* the maintenance rate *plus* an additional one-half of the maintenance rate.

The child's response to crystalloid replacement should be monitored by assessing the child's intake and output. In particular, normal urine output should be approximately 1 mL/kg per hour. If the child is oliguric, then the child still may be dehydrated. Likewise, a urine specific gravity in excess of 1.030 may suggest dehydration. Daily weights should be assessed as a measure of fluid balance rather than loss or gain of lean body mass. A sudden gain or loss of weight in a dehydrated child is related most commonly to fluid gains or losses.[52]

BLOOD COMPONENTS

The same indications for delivery of blood components in adults that were outlined in Chapter 9 are indications for transfusion of various blood components in infants and children. Because of their smaller size, however, infants and children are most likely to receive split packs of blood components. Use of split packs means that children will receive only specified milliliters of blood components rather than full units. Furthermore, because infants and children tend to have immature immune systems compared with adults, they are more likely to receive split packs of modified packed red blood cells (PRBCs) than their adult counterparts.[52] These modified PRBCs may be irradiated, washed, leukocyte-reduced, or specially screened for cytomegalovirus (CMV). Descriptions of methods to modify PRBCs and their respective specific indications were noted in Chapter 9.

PARENTERAL NUTRITION

The methods to deliver parenteral nutrients to infants and children are very similar to those discussed for adults in Chapter 10. In general, infants and children have higher metabolic demands than adults and hence have heightened nutritional requirements. Because of this, peripheral parenteral nutrition (PPN) is indicated for use in infants and children only rarely.[52]

MEDICATION

The methods advocated to deliver I.V. medications to infants and children mirror those in adults, with the obvious additional caveat that infants and children require smaller dosages of medications and solutions. Chapter 11 presents general guidelines for the delivery of I.V. medications.

Summary

There are important physiologic and psychological differences that characterize the different stages of development among infants and children. The nurse who cares for infants and children for whom I.V. therapy is prescribed must master basic minimal competencies in the care of infants and children. This chapter specifies some key differences between the developmental stage of infants and children and among infants, children, and adults that affect the delivery of I.V. therapy. However, it is beyond the scope of this book to provide comprehensive pediatric-specific

I.V. therapy guidelines. Nurses who care for infants and children are encouraged to find supplemental pediatric-specific I.V. therapy resources that can guide their practice.

Quiz

1. A child who is 5 years of age and who weighs 14 kg is considered to belong to which developmental stage?

    (a) Infancy

    (b) Toddler

    (c) Preschool

    (d) School-aged

2. Infusion sets indicated for use among infants and children are characterized by which of the following?

    (a) Lack of a spike to access the I.V. container

    (b) A minidrop chamber that produces 50–60 drops/mL

    (c) Large-volume delivery chambers

    (d) Intravenous pumps that are programmed to deliver large volumes

3. Minimum competencies that must be mastered by the nurse who delivers I.V. therapy to infants and children include all but which of the following?

    (a) Competency in finding appropriate vascular access sites in infants and children

    (b) Cognizance of the physiologic differences between infants and children who represent different developmental stages

    (c) Cognizance of the psychological differences between infants and children who represent different developmental stages

    (d) Competence in working with generic I.V. therapy equipment

4. A key disadvantage to the application of topical anesthetic creams prior to gaining I.V. access is that they

    (a) take at least 1 hour to be effective.

    (b) do not work equally effectively with children who represent each developmental stage.

(c) are expensive.

(d) are volatile.

5. Which of the following statements concerning indications to access scalp veins for delivering I.V. therapy is *true*?

   (a) Scalp veins are readily accessible in infants and children who represent all developmental stages.

   (b) When scalp veins are accessed, the tip of the needle should be pointed downward, towards the patient's chest.

   (c) Scalp veins are less prone to adverse events such as infiltration than other peripheral veins.

   (d) Scalp veins are a first-line choice for gaining peripheral I.V. access in infants.

6. A child who weights 15 kg and who is mildly dehydrated should receive how many milliliters of crystalloids during the first 24 hours of I.V. therapy?

   (a) 1000 mL

   (b) 1250 mL

   (c) 1875 mL

   (d) 2500 mL

7. Infants and children are more likely to receive modified packs of packed red blood cells (PRBCs) than adults because

   (a) they are more prone to fluid overload than adults.

   (b) they are more prone to electrolyte disturbances than adults.

   (c) they are more prone to fluid shifts than adults.

   (d) they are more prone to immune-related dysfunction than adults.

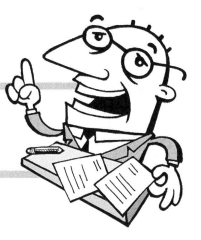

CHAPTER 13

Intravenous Therapy and the Older Adult

Learning Objectives

After completing this chapter, the learner will

1   Identify different age groups of older adults.

2   Describe differences in intravenous (I.V.) delivery systems and I.V. access devices that are indicated for use in older adults from those indicated for use in younger adults.

3   Recognize basic competencies that must be mastered by nurses who administer I.V. therapy to older adults.

4   Identify an alternate infusion access site that might be used in older adults.

5   Discuss guidelines for administration of I.V. crystalloids, blood components, parenteral nutrients, and medications in older adults.

Key Terms

Older adult   Oldest old
Young old   Venous sclerosis
Middle old   Hypodermoclysis

Indications for Intravenous (I.V.) Therapy in Older Adults

Indications for I.V. therapy in older adults mirror those for other age groups. Intravenous therapy in older adults is indicated to achieve or maintain fluid and electrolyte balance, replace or supplement needed blood components, provide nutrients, and administer medications. The term **older adult** generally refers to those who are 65 years of age or older,[57] although there is no clear consensus on this age classification. For instance, traumatologists note that adults 55 years of age and older generally respond to interventions indicated to treat traumatic injuries in a different manner than younger adults, and therefore, they tend to classify these younger-aged adults as older adults.

1 Older adults are sometimes classified based on their age groups. Older adults may be considered **young old** if they are between 65 and 74 years of age, **middle old** if they are between 75 and 84 years of age, and old old or **oldest old** if they are at least 85 years of age.[57,58] These classifications are not used to guide specific I.V. therapy initiation or maintenance regimens among different age groups of older adults. Nonetheless, it is generally acknowledged that it is harder to gain I.V. access and initiate and maintain I.V. therapy in oldest old adults than in young old or middle old adults.

Older adults receive I.V. therapy more commonly than any other age group. In the United States, adults 65 years of age and older account for almost half the hospitalizations as well as almost half of all hospital days, approximately 80 percent of all home health care visits, and approximately 90 percent of all long-term-care facility placements.[59,60] Some of the most common reasons to initiate I.V. therapy among older adults are to treat dehydration and correct electrolyte imbalances, to administer I.V. antibiotics, and to administer chemotherapeutic agents.

SPEED BUMP

_____ *receive I.V. therapy more commonly than any other age group.*

This chapter provides a cursory overview of some of the basic principles of administering I.V. therapy in older adults. The reader is encouraged to review additional sources of information to find more specific and comprehensive content on I.V. therapy and older adults.

Selecting I.V. Therapy Delivery Systems for Older Adults ②

INFUSION SETS

Intravenous line sets used in older adults tend to be the same as those used in other age groups. Some frail older adults may not be able to tolerate the same volumes of fluids, blood components, nutrients, and medications that are indicated in other, healthier adults. In particular, older adults with a known history of heart or renal failure may require lower rates of infusion or may suffer fluid overload. In these cases, the I.V. administration sets must be capable of delivering lesser amounts of solution. Sometimes smaller I.V. containers (i.e., I.V. bottles and bags) are hung. In other instances, the primary infusion set selected may be the same set used in pediatric patients, that is, a minidrop infusion set or an I.V. set with a volume-limited chamber.[57] These infusion sets are described in Chapter 12.

ELECTRONIC INFUSION DEVICES

All older adults should receive I.V. therapy by electronic infusion devices, also called *I.V. pumps.* Older adults are much more susceptible to the adverse effects of volume overload than younger adults, even those without a known history of cardiovascular or renal disease. In general, I.V. pumps that are used for delivering I.V. fluids to younger adults are indicated to deliver I.V. fluids to older adults as well because they can be programmed to deliver small volumes of fluid reliably and accurately. Chapter 3 provides a description of I.V. pumps.

Patient Preparation

Prior to initiating I.V. therapy, the nurse must verify that an appropriate prescriptive order has been written by a physician or other advanced-practice clinician recognized by the respective state board of nursing as having the authority to prescribe this type of interventional therapy. Authorized advanced-practice clinicians may include nurse practitioners, nurse midwives, nurse anesthetists, or physician assistants. In general, the preparatory guidelines outlined in Chapters 4 and 5 as appropriate for adult patients who are slated to begin I.V. therapy by either peripheral or central I.V. access routes are also appropriate for older adults.[6] Informed consent should be obtained from the older adult patient prior to initiating I.V. therapy.[6]

3 The nurse who is responsible for initiating I.V. therapy in older adults must master certain competencies. The nurse should be

- Comfortable and competent in finding and accessing appropriate vascular access routes in older adults

- Cognizant of the physiologic, sensory, and cognitive differences between adults and older adults

- Comfortable and competent in working with I.V. therapy and understanding its interactive effects with multiple other therapies that the older adult may be receiving[6]

Peripheral I.V. Therapy

SELECTION OF VASCULAR ACCESS SITES

Selection of peripheral I.V. access sites in older adults tends to follow the general guidelines for younger adults noted in Chapter 4. The same veins that are preferred access sites in younger adults are preferred access sites in older adults. However, gaining vascular access may be more difficult in the older adult because the veins are more fragile, particularly if the older adult has significant comorbid conditions or represents the oldest old age group.

As older adults continue to age, they progressively lose more skeletal muscle mass, and the veins become progressively more sclerotic. The loss of muscle mass in older adults has the effect of making their veins less stable, and they "roll" when they are accessed by an I.V. needle (i.e., when venipuncture is performed). **Venous sclerosis** has the effect of making the veins stiffer and more fragile, which may result in quicker I.V. infiltration than is otherwise typical. In addition, sclerosed veins tend to have narrower lumens than healthier veins, which further challenges successful I.V. access with a venous access device.

SPEED BUMP

Older adults commonly have veins that are stiffer, more fragile, and with narrower lumens, a phenomenon called venous _____.

In older adults who are either oldest old or who have significant comorbidities, it is frequently advisable to forego trying to access the veins on the dorsum of the hand. Loss of muscle mass on the hands and venous sclerosis can make access of these veins particularly challenging. Loss of muscle mass on the forearms also can make those veins less stable. Placing slight traction on the accessed vein at sites slightly distal and proximal to the venipuncture site may help to stabilize the vein and prevent it from rolling. This may be accomplished by using the thumb and forefinger of the hand used to hold the patient's forearm to apply a slight amount of pulling pressure in opposing directions on either end of the vein.

The nurse should carefully palpate any vein that may be a candidate for I.V. access to confirm that the vein feels supple and pliable. Veins that feel stiff and tortuous might become infiltrated shortly after access with an I.V. needle, before the catheter can be fully advanced. Eliminating the use of a tourniquet or minimizing the time that the tourniquet is applied so that the vessel is less engorged with blood and there is less pressure in the vessel when it is accessed might be an effective method to ensure successful placement of an I.V. access device in an older adult.[57]

SELECTION OF VASCULAR ACCESS DEVICES

The same types of vascular access devices used in younger adults also can be used in older adults. These include steel-winged infusion devices and short and midline over-the-needle catheters, which were described in Chapter 4. Older adults generally require smaller-gauge catheters and needles than are used in their younger-adult counterparts partly because the lumens of their veins narrow from age-related venous sclerosis.[57]

Central I.V. Therapy

SELECTION OF VASCULAR ACCESS SITES

Selection of central I.V. access sites in older adults mirrors that in younger adults and was described in Chapter 5. As is true with peripheral I.V. therapy, gaining vascular access may be more difficult in the older adult, however, because the veins are more fragile.

SELECTION OF VASCULAR ACCESS DEVICES

Vascular access devices that are appropriate for gaining central I.V. access in older adults are similar to those used in younger adults but tend to have smaller lumens to better accommodate the narrower venous lumens of older adults. Chapter 5 discusses the sizes and characteristics of a number of central vascular access devices.

Alternative Infusion Therapy Delivery Sites ④

HYPODERMOCLYSIS

Hypodermoclysis refers to the administration of crystalloids into the subcutaneous space. This type of infusion therapy is indicated most frequently in frail older adults who are residents of long-term care facilities and who are suffering from mild or moderate dehydration. It is sometimes indicated for terminally ill patients with mild or moderate dehydration who are expected to recover from the effects of dehydration with the administration of these fluids or for terminally ill patients as a means to deliver opioids and sedatives.[61]

Preferred sites for administering fluids by this method are those with adequate deposits of subcutaneous tissue. Although the most common site used is the lower abdomen, the thighs and the outer aspect of the upper arms also may be used. Any type of needle that is no longer than 1 inch may be used to gain access to the subcutaneous tissue. The needle is attached to a typical I.V. administration setup. The most common crystalloids administered in this way include 0.9% or 0.45% saline. Fluid may be delivered at a rate that does not exceed 1 mL/minute or more than 3000 mL in 24 hours.[16,61] Hypodermoclysis is not associated with some of the common adverse events associated with I.V. therapy, such as fluid overload, phlebitis, thrombosis, and sepsis, but fluid absorption may be less than optimal with hypodermoclysis, and access-site edema occurs commonly.

Delivery of I.V. Therapy in Older Adults ⑤

CRYSTALLOIDS

The most common indications for initiating I.V. therapy in older adults are to either treat or prevent a disruption in fluid and electrolytes. In general, the same principles that generally guide the delivery of crystalloids noted in Chapter 7 guide the infusion of crystalloids in older adults. However, older adults are much more susceptible to fluid overload than their younger counterparts, even those without a known history of cardiovascular or renal disease. The general adage in replenishing fluids and electrolytes in older adults is to "start low and go slow." That is, initiation of I.V. therapy in older adults generally should commence at a lower rate than in their younger counterparts, a rate that may be titrated upward gradually as the older adult demonstrates tolerance of the fluids administered.

The older adult's response to crystalloid replacement should be monitored by assessing intake and output. In particular, normal urine output in an older adult should be at least 0.5 mL/kg per hour and optimally 1.0 mL/kg per hour. Daily weights should be assessed as a measure of fluid balance rather than loss or gain of lean body mass. A sudden gain or loss of weight in an acutely ill older adult is related most commonly to fluid gains or losses. Assessing the older adult's baseline heart and lung sounds prior to initiating I.V. therapy is a good practice. Clinical signs and symptoms seen after I.V. therapy is begun that might indicate fluid overload include the new presence of

- Bibasilar crackles

- Productive cough, particularly if the sputum is frothy and pink-tinged

- Dyspnea

- An S_3

- A murmur or increased grade of a previous murmur

- Oliguria

If any of these manifestations of fluid overload are noted, the physician should be notified, and the worrisome signs and symptoms should be noted in the patient's record. The I.V. infusion rate likely will be decreased, and the patient might be treated with I.V. diuretics.

BLOOD COMPONENTS

The same indications for delivery of blood components in younger adults that were outlined in Chapter 9 are indications for transfusions of blood components in older adults. Older adults are more likely to manifest volume overload than their younger-adult counterparts, however. Because of this, older adults may be prescribed split packs of blood components, which contain fractions of full units. In addition, because more older adult patients may have received multiple blood transfusions previously, and because more older adult patients are immunosuppressed because of their higher rates of autoimmune disorders and cancers, they are more likely to receive modified packed red blood cells (PRBCs) than their younger-adult counterparts.[52] These modified

PRBCs may be irradiated, washed, leukocyte-reduced, or specially screened for cytomegalovirus (CMV). Descriptions of methods to modify PRBCs and their respective specific indications are noted in Chapter 9.

PARENTERAL NUTRITION

The methods to deliver parenteral nutrients to older adults mirror those for younger adults and were outlined in Chapter 10. In general, older adults are more likely to be undernourished or malnourished than younger adults[58] and are more commonly candidates for parenteral nutrition therapy.

MEDICATION

The methods advocated to deliver I.V. medications to older adults are the same as those advocated to deliver I.V. medications to younger adults. However, there are certain considerations that should be noted whenever I.V. medications are administered to older adults. These include that

- Older adult patients are more likely to be prescribed multiple medications. Adverse interaction effects that occur from administering multiple medications therefore are more likely to occur in older adult patients than in other patients.

- The older the adult, the lower is the glomerular filtration rate, and the less effective the kidneys are at excreting by-products of drugs cleared through the kidneys. Therefore, the effects of drugs and their metabolic by-products that are normally cleared through the kidneys tend to linger longer in older adult patients.

- The older the adult, the less effective the liver becomes at metabolizing drugs. Therefore, the effects of drugs that are normally metabolized through the liver linger longer in older adult patients.

- The older the adult, the less is the lean skeletal mass, and the serum albumin level may decrease proportionately. Drugs that normally bind to albumin may be less bound when administered, and the effects of those drugs may be greater.

Given each of these caveats, older adults who receive I.V. medications generally should receive these medications more cautiously than their younger-adult counterparts.[60,62,63] The adage to "start low and go slow" certainly applies to titration of I.V. medications among older adult patients. It is advisable to consult with pharmacists whenever older adult patients who either have significant comorbidities or who are prescribed multiple medications are prescribed I.V. medications so that therapy can be optimally guided.

Summary

There are important guidelines to the safe and effective delivery of I.V. therapy in older adults that are different from those in their younger-adult counterparts. Since older adults represent the age group that is the most common recipient of I.V. therapy, the nurse who cares for older adults must master basic minimal competencies in delivering I.V. therapy to older adults. Nurses who routinely care for older adults who receive I.V. therapy are encouraged to find supplemental gerontology-specific I.V. therapy resources that can guide their practice.

Quiz

1. The group of older adults who comprise the oldest age group (e.g., ≥85 years of age) are referred to as the

    (a) gerontologic set.

    (b) young old.

    (c) middle old.

    (d) oldest old.

2. A common complication that occurs from administering high volumes of I.V. fluids to older adults is

    (a) fluid overload.

    (b) dehydration.

    (c) delirium.

    (d) chronic renal failure.

3. Veins that should be considered first for peripheral I.V. access in older adults include

    (a) veins of the dorsum of the hand.

    (b) the subclavian vein.

    (c) the femoral vein.

    (d) the veins of the forearm.

4. Methods that may help to ensure successful peripheral venous access in the older adult include all but which of the following?

(a) Applying light traction to the accessed vein at points distal and proximal to the venipuncture access site

(b) Minimizing the time that a tourniquet is applied

(c) Selecting a venous access site that is tortuous and is at a point of a bifurcation

(d) Palpating a vein to ensure that it is supple and pliable before it is selected as a suitable site

5. Sites that may be selected for hypodermoclysis include

(a) the same sites that are suitable for peripheral I.V. access.

(b) the same sites that are suitable for central I.V. access.

(c) the lower abdomen.

(d) the external jugular vein.

6. Clinical manifestations of fluid overload may include all but which of the following?

(a) Bibasilar crackles

(b) Thrombophlebitis

(c) Dyspnea

(d) Oliguria

7. An older adult patient who is prescribed I.V. digoxin (Lanoxin) is severely hypoalbuminemic. Digoxin is bound to albumin in the plasma. The nurse knows that which of the following statements is *true*?

(a) The patient should receive lesser than typical doses of I.V. digoxin because the patient could have the adverse effect of digoxin toxicity.

(b) The patient should receive higher than typical doses of I.V. digoxin because the patient might not reap the therapeutic effects of digoxin.

(c) The patient should receive normally prescribed doses of digoxin because its binding with serum albumin should have no effect on its toxicity.

(d) The patient should receive normally prescribed doses of digoxin because its binding with serum albumin should have no effect on its therapeutic effectiveness.

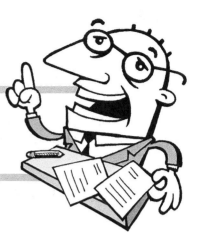

CHAPTER 14

Intravenous Therapy within Community-Based Settings

Learning Objectives

After completing this chapter, the learner will

1. Identify community-based settings where intravenous (I.V) therapy may be delivered.

2. Describe the role of the nurse in delivering I.V. therapy within community-based settings.

3 Recognize the nurse's role in teaching patients and families how to maintain I.V. access sites safely and effectively within community-based settings.

4 Recognize the nurse's role in teaching patients and families how to self-administer I.V. therapy safely and effectively within home-based settings.

 Key Terms

Community-based settings

Introduction to Community-Based Settings

Much of this book focuses on the delivery of I.V. therapy within the confines of the hospital. However, I.V. therapy may be delivered in a variety of community-based settings outside the hospital. Administering I.V. therapy in settings outside the hospital tends to cost less and gives patients more freedom, which can enhance patient quality of life. Within this context, **community-based settings** refer to therapy that is delivered to patients and families who reside within the confines of an identifiable geographic region. **1** Some of the community-based settings where I.V. therapy may be delivered include

- Clinics that are either hospital-based or freestanding
- Infusion therapy centers
- Ambulatory-care centers, including same-day surgery centers, diagnostic facilities, and urgent-care centers
- Long-term care facilities
- Hospices
- Assisted-living facilities[64]
- Traditional home settings[65]

When a patient receives I.V. therapy within the traditional home setting, the person who administers the I.V. therapy may be the patient or a home health care nurse. This chapter provides a brief overview of some basic principles for administering I.V. therapy within community-based settings, including the home setting. The reader is encouraged to review additional sources of information to find more specific and comprehensive content on I.V. therapy within specific community-based settings.

Speed Bump

_____ *refer to therapy that is delivered to patients and families who reside within the confines of an identifiable geographic region.*

The Role of the Nurse in Delivering I.V. Therapy within Community-Based Settings

2 The nurse who administers I.V. therapy within community-based settings may be responsible for initiating the administration of I.V. infusions. If this is the case, the same principles that guide selection and setup of I.V. delivery systems that were discussed in Chapter 3 also apply to community-based settings. The nurse who practices in a same-day surgery center may be responsible for initiating multiple peripheral I.V. setups for patients on a daily basis. In this event, the principles that guide selection of peripheral access sites and venous access devices that were outlined in Chapter 4 can be applied to this setting. The nurse who works in an oncology clinic and who administers cyclic infusions of chemotherapeutic agents to cancer patients with central venous access devices may use the principles outlined in Chapter 5. Likewise, the same principles that guide general nursing practice noted in Chapter 6 and that guide the appropriate infusion of crystalloid solutions (e.g., Chapter 7), colloid solutions (e.g., Chapter 8), blood components (e.g., Chapter 9), parenteral nutrition (e.g., Chapter 10), and medications (e.g., Chapter 11) and special populations such as infants and children (e.g., Chapter 12) and older adults (e.g., Chapter 13) can be used as general guides for the administration of I.V. therapy to patients within community-based settings.

PATIENT AND FAMILY TEACHING NEEDS

Patients who receive I.V. therapy within community-based settings do not fit a single profile. Often patients who present to ambulatory-care centers who require I.V. therapy have diagnostic procedures performed (e.g., colonoscopies) or same-day surgical procedures (e.g., tonsillectomies). These patients receive I.V. push or bolus dosages of anesthetics and anxiolytic agents by peripheral venous access routes that are initiated and discontinued within a few hours. Patients such as these who require I.V. therapy for brief time periods and who have limited responsibility for maintaining I.V. access have limited teaching needs about their therapy.

Many patients who receive I.V. therapy within community-based settings receive either cyclic or continuous infusions to treat chronic diseases. Because the

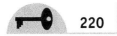
anticipated time frame for the delivery of I.V. therapy is longer than a few days, these patients require the placement of some type of central venous access device, which may include a peripherally inserted central catheter (PICC), a nontunneled catheter, a tunneled catheter, or an implantable port. Patients who require this type of therapy may include any of the following:

- Patients with chronic infections (e.g., patients with osteomyelitis; hepatic, splenic, or brain abscesses; septic arthritis or bursitis; chronic complicated sinusitis; otitis media; or mastoiditis) who require cyclic doses of a variety of I.V. antibiotics

- Patients with cancer who require cyclic doses of a variety of chemotherapeutic agents

- Patients who are undernourished or malnourished and who require continuous or cyclic I.V. infusions of parenteral nutrition

- Patients with heart failure who require cyclic doses of I.V. inotropic agents (e.g., dobutamine)

- Patients with pulmonary arterial hypertension who require continuous infusions of epoprostenol (Flolan)

Patients with Central Venous Access Devices

3 Patients with central venous access devices and their family members who are either primary caregivers or who share some of the caretaking responsibilities must understand how to maintain the central venous access devices so that they do not experience access-related adverse events. They must be taught methods to ensure asepsis of the venous access site, and they must be taught the manifestations of venous access-site-related adverse events. In addition, any patient with a central venous access device who is not a hospital inpatient should be told to wear a medical alert bracelet. In the event of an emergency, health care providers could have ready access to a central I.V. line if necessary or may be alerted that manipulation of the central I.V. access device is contraindicated if the patient wears an appropriate medical alert bracelet.

SPEED BUMP

Patients and family members within community-based settings who have central venous access devices for the delivery of I.V. therapy must be taught methods to ensure _____ of the venous access site, and they must be taught manifestations of venous access-site-related adverse events.

Patients with central venous access devices and their family members must be taught how to maintain their devices properly to minimize the likelihood of contamination. In particular, they must be

- Taught how to cover their access-site dressings when they shower or bathe so that the dressings do not become wet.
- Given checklists of supplies that they must keep on hand to change their dressings.
- Taught about the importance of handwashing prior to changing the dressing.
- Taught when to change the dressings, that is, every 7 days for dressings with transparent semipermeable membranes or on contamination.
- Taught how to change their dressings and cleanse their access sites. In order to ensure that these patients and families members are capable of performing these skills, the nurse also should give readily understandable instruction sheets on venous access-site care to these patients and family members as resource guides and ask them to perform return demonstrations to show that they truly understand what needs to be done and have mastered the psychomotor skills needed to change the dressings and cleanse the access sites.

Patients with central venous access devices and their family members also must be taught to monitor for clinical manifestations of central venous access-site-related adverse events. These include the following:

- Sepsis, which may be manifested by fever, lethargy, chills, or shock symptoms
- Access-site infection, which may be manifested by fever, redness, swelling, or purulent drainage at the venous access site
- Phlebitis, which may be manifested by redness, swelling, or a burning sensation at the venous access site
- Thrombosis, which may be manifested by an inability to infuse either flush solution or other solutions into the venous access device
- Air embolism, which may be manifested by sudden dyspnea, disorientation, diaphoresis, or shock symptoms

These patients and their families must be taught to report any suspicions of adverse events to their health care provider. In particular, patients who may be manifesting sepsis or air embolism should be taught how to appropriately seek immediate emergency care. A list of phone numbers to call if any of these adverse events occur should be readily available.

Self-Administration of I.V. Therapy

Some patients who require long-term I.V. therapy either self-administer or have family members help them administer their infusions within their homes. In some cases, these infusions are continuous, whereas in other cases, they are cyclic. Not only must the patients and their family members be screened in advance to ensure that they have the cognitive and psychomotor abilities to safely deliver the I.V. therapy as prescribed, the home environment also must be screened in advance. The home environment must be clean, must have running hot water, must have a ready source of electricity to provide power to charge the I.V. pump batteries, and must have a telephone line so that emergency calls can be made as needed. In some cases, a clean refrigerator may be needed to store the I.V. infusions, which may include I.V. medications or I.V. parenteral nutrition solutions.

    4 Patients and any family members who are caregivers must be taught how to maintain the infusions safely and effectively. The nurse should provide these patients and caregivers with formal instruction, give them readily understandable written guidelines, and critique return demonstrations of psychomotor skills to ensure that they are mastered appropriately. Patients and family members must be given appropriate phone numbers to call in event of questions, equipment malfunction, or emergencies. Not only must they be able to demonstrate the ability to change their dressings and cleanse their I.V. access sites, but they also must be able to

- Discuss the characteristics of the I.V. infusion and why it is prescribed
- Identify any side effects, toxic effects, or adverse effects associated with delivery of the I.V. infusion and how to respond if they occur
- Demonstrate appropriate handling (e.g., refrigeration and temperature control) of the I.V. infusion
- Demonstrate appropriate use and handling of the I.V. infusion pump
- Demonstrate how to set up and prime the I.V. administration set
- Demonstrate how to connect and disconnect the I.V. administration set from the venous access site
- Demonstrate how to flush the I.V. venous access site so that it remains patent

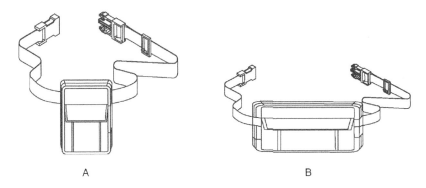

Figure 14-1   Accessories for ambulatory I.V. pumps. *A.* Small, soft fanny pack (50–100 mL). *B.* Large, soft fanny pack (250–1000 mL). (Courtesy of B. Braun, Products Catalog, 2005.)

Many patients who self-administer I.V. therapy at home do so using I.V. administration sets that do not differ from those described previously in this book. The electronic infusion devices (i.e., I.V. pumps) that are used, however, tend to be much smaller in size than those used in the hospital-based setting. These ambulatory or portable I.V. pumps feature the same essential capabilities as their larger counterparts but do allow the home care patient more flexibility in ambulation. These pumps can be battery-charged and then placed in a "fanny pack" that the patient can wear. Figure 14-1 shows fanny packs that can hold either small or larg I.V. bags.

Summary

Patients who receive I.V. therapy are not necessarily confined to the hospital setting. Delivering I.V. therapy to patients within community-based settings can be more cost-effective and can enhance patients' quality of life. There are a number of community-based settings where I.V. therapy may be administered. Patients with central venous access devices must be able to maintain these sites safely for continued delivery of their prescribed I.V. infusions. Patients and their families who self-administer I.V. infusions within the home setting must live in an appropriate environment that supports the safe and effective delivery of their prescribed therapy. Furthermore, they must demonstrate the psychomotor skills necessary to deliver their I.V. infusions safely and effectively.

Quiz

1. Community-based settings where I.V. therapy may be administered include all but which of the following?

   (a) Same-day surgery centers

   (b) Hospices

   (c) Inpatient rehabilitation units

   (d) Infusion-therapy centers

2. Patients who receive I.V. therapy within community-based settings with the most limited teaching needs include those who receive their infusions within

   (a) same-day surgery centers.

   (b) hospices.

   (c) inpatient rehabilitation units.

   (d) infusion-therapy centers.

3. Chronic diseases that may warrant either cyclic or continuous I.V. therapy over the long term within community-based settings include all but which of the following?

   (a) Heart failure

   (b) Appendicitis

   (c) Cancer

   (d) Osteomyelitis

4. Patients who have central I.V. access devices and their families should be taught

   (a) how to prevent venous access-site sepsis.

   (b) how to self-administer all their infusions.

   (c) how to treat an air embolism.

   (d) how to dissolve an access-site thrombus.

5. The home environment for patients eligible to self-administer their I.V. infusions must be

(a) on one level.

(b) within 5 miles of the primary infusion center.

(c) in a neighborhood that is relatively safe to accommodate home care visits.

(d) clean.

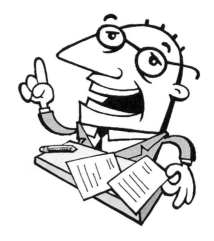

Answers to Quiz Questions

Chapter 1: Introduction to Intravenous Therapy

1. a. Intravenous
2. c. Alimentary
3. c. Infusion Nurses Certification Corporation
4. c. Treating dehydration
5. a. ABO blood types
6. b. Gastric infusion

Chapter 2: Fluids and Electrolytes

1. b. A normal-sized, healthy adult male
2. a. Intracellular
3. d. Albumin

4. b.   Osmosis

5. a.   Sodium

6. c.   Hypertonic

7. b.   Metabolic acidosis

8. a.   No more than 10 mEq/h in an admixed solution. If a central I.V. line is used, no more than 20 mEq/h.

9. d.   Hypocalcemia treatment

Chapter 3: Intravenous Therapy Delivery Systems

1. c.   Luer-lock connections.

2. d.   They tend to be compatible with medications and solutions that interact with plastics.

3. d.   Intravenous tubing.

4. d.   50 drops/mL

5. b.   125 mL/h

6. b.   125 mL/h

7. d.   750 mL/h

8. b.   30 drops/minute

9. d.   42 drops/minute

10. a.   17 drops/minute

11. c.   60 drops/minute

12. d.   67 drops/minute

13. a.   33 drops/minute

14. b.   50 drops/minute

15. a.   Feature a variety of alarms

Chapter 4: Peripheral Intravenous Therapy

1. d.   To provide parenteral nutrition

2. b.   A nontortuous metacarpal vein on a nondominant hand

3. a.   A steel winged-tipped infusion device

4. c.   Whenever the system is contaminated

5. c.   The catheter

6. c.   Whenever they are soiled

Chapter 5: Central Intravenous Therapy

1. a.   PICC

2. a.   Basilic

3. b.   Subclavian

4. d.   Infiltration

5. b.   Air embolism

Chapter 6: Intravenous Therapy and the Nursing Process

1. d.   Decreased cardiac output

2. b.   Patients with dry mucus membranes

3. d.   Purulent drainage

4. a.   Infiltration

5. a.   Disuse syndrome may be prevented by choosing a peripheral access site that is not in close proximity to a joint.

Chapter 7: Crystalloid Solutions

1. b.   Isotonic solutions

2. a.   Saline (0.9% NS)

3. b.   An isotonic solution

4. a.   A hypotonic solution

5. c.   125 mL

6. a.   375 mL

7. d.   None

8. c.   Hypertonic

9. c.   The blood cells and vascular endothelial cells shrink when they come into contact with the solution.

10. c.   501 mL

11. d.   999 mL

12. a.   The blood cells and vascular endothelial cells are not affected by coming in contact with the solution.

13. a.   0 mL of solution disperses into the intracellular space, 375 mL of solution disperses to the interstitium, and 125 mL of solution remains in the intravascular space.

Chapter 8: Colloid Solutions

1. b.   Colloids pass readily through capillary and cell membranes.

2. a.   Plasma protein fraction

3. c.   Leukapharesis

4. b.   Carbohydrate macromolecules

5. d.   Dextran

6. d.   Dextran

Chapter 9: Blood Component Therapy

1. a.   15 g/dL

2. c.   Recombinant granulocyte-colony stimulating factor (G-CSF)

3. d.   42 days after it is donated

4. b.   3 percent

5. a.   Preoperative autologous blood donation (PABD)

6. c.   Leukocyte-reduced

7. c.   All patients with platelet counts <10,000/mm^3

8. d.   Patients receiving warfarin (Coumadin) who require quick reversal of its anticoagulation effects

9. a.   Type A

10. c.   Type AB

11. d. Women of childbearing years

12. d. All the above

13. a. Acute hemolytic reaction

14. b. Febrile nonhemolytic reaction

15. d. Must use secure Luer-lock connections, as appropriate

Chapter 10: Parenteral Nutrition Therapy

1. d. A patient with a bowel obstruction

2. c. A patient who is prescribed warfarin (Coumadin)

3. c. Total nutrient admixture (TNA)

4. d. I.V. fat emulsion (IVFE)

5. a. Continuous

6. b. Ondansetron (Zofran)

7. c. Hyperglycemia

8. d. Refeeding syndrome

Chapter 11: Intravenous Pharmacologic Therapy

1. b. Quick drug action can be ensured only by administering the medication intravenously.

2. b. Medications maintain their stability long after their expiration date and still may be given intravenously.

3. b. The patient's room number

4. a. Extravasation

5. b. 100 mL/h

6. d. A cognitively intact and otherwise healthy 30-year-old man who is postoperative after donating a kidney to his brother

7. a. Stop the infusion

8. b. Potentiated

Chapter 12: Intravenous Therapy and Infants and Children

1. c.   Preschool

2. b.   A minidrop chamber of 50–60 drops/mL

3. d.   Competence in working with generic I.V. therapy equipment

4. a.   Take at least 1 hour to be effective

5. b.   When scalp veins are accessed, the tip of the needle should be pointed downward, toward the patient's chest.

6. c.   1875 mL

7. d.   They are more prone to immune-related dysfunction than adults.

Chapter 13: Intravenous Therapy and the Older Adult

1. d.   Oldest old

2. a.   Fluid overload

3. d.   The veins of the forearm

4. c.   Selecting a venous access site that is tortuous and that is at a point of a bifurcation

5. c.   The lower abdomen

6. b.   Thrombophlebitis

7. a.   The patient should receive lesser than typical doses of I.V. digoxin (Lanoxin) or the patient could have the adverse effect of digoxin toxicity.

Chapter 14: Intravenous Therapy within Community-Based Settings

1. c.   Inpatient rehabilitation units

2. a.   Same-day surgery centers

3. b.   Appendicitis

4. a.   How to prevent venous access-site sepsis

5. d.   Clean

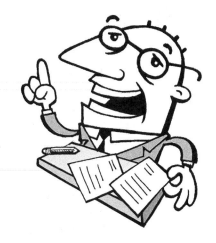

References

1. Sandelowski M: Venous envy: The post-World War II debate over IV nursing. *Adv Nurs Sci* 22:56–62, 1999.
2. Corrigan AM: History of intravenous therapy. In Hankins J, Lonsway RA, Hedrick C, et al. (eds.): *Infusion Therapy in Clinical Practice,* 2nd ed. Philadelphia: Saunders, 2001.
3. Cosnett JE: The origins of intravenous fluid therapy. *Lancet* 1:768–771, 1989.
4. Sheehy TW: Origins of intravenous fluid therapy. *Lancet* 1:1081, 1989.
5. Cheever KH: Early enteral feeding of the multitrauma patient. *Crit Care Nurse* 19:40–51, 1999.
6. Infusion Nurses Society: Infusion nursing: Standards of practice. *J Infus Nurs* 28:S1–S77, 2006.
7. Infusion Nurses Certification Corporation: http://ins.trprod-development.com/certification/index.html; accessed on January 10, 2007.
8. Matkin G, Porth CM: Disorders of fluid and electrolyte balance. In Porth CM (ed.): *Pathophysiology: Concepts of Altered Health States,* 7th ed. Philadelphia: Lippincott Williams & Wilkins, 2005.
9. Edwards S: Regulation of water, sodium and potassium: Implications for practice. *Nurs Standard* 15:36–45, 2001.

10. Allison S: Fluid, electrolytes and nutrition. *Scand J Nutr* 47:99–102, 2003.
11. Hankins J: The role of albumin in fluid and electrolyte balance. *J Infus Nurs* 29:260–265, 2006.
12. Metheny NM: *Fluid and Electrolyte Balance: Nursing Considerations.* Philadelphia: Lippincott Williams & Wilkins, 2000.
13. Elgart HN: Assessment of fluids and electrolytes. *AACN Clin Issues* 15:607–621, 2004.
14. Burger CM: Hypokalemia: Averting crisis with early recognition and intervention. *Am J Nurs* 104:61–65, 2004.
15. Burger CM: Hyperkalemia: When serum K^+ is not okay. *Am J Nurs* 104:66–70, 2004.
16. Perucca R: Infusion therapy equipment: Types of infusion therapy equipment. In Hankins J, Lonsway RAW, Hedrick C, Perdue MB (eds.): *The Infusion Nurses Society: Infusion Therapy in Clinical Practice,* 2nd ed. Philadelphia: Saunders, 2001.
17. Perucca R: Obtaining vascular access. In Hankins J, Lonsway RAW, Hedrick C, Perdue MB (eds.): *The Infusion Nurses Society: Infusion Therapy in Clinical Practice,* 2nd ed. Philadelphia: Saunders, 2001.
18. NANDA: *Nursing Diagnoses: Definitions & Classification 2005–2006.* Philadelphia: NANDA International, 2005.
19. Johnson M, Bulecheck G, Dochterman J, et al.: *Nursing Diagnoses, Outcomes, & Interventions: NANDA, NOC, and NIC Linkages.* St. Louis, MO: Elsevier, 2006.
20. Cook LS: IV fluid resuscitation. *J Infus Nurs* 26:296–303, 2003.
21. Kelley CM: Hypovolemic shock: An overview. *Crit Care Nurs Q* 28:2–19, 2005.
22. Hankins J, Hedrik C: Parenteral fluids. In Hankins J, Lonsway RA, Hedrick C, et al. (eds.): *Infusion Therapy in Clinical Practice,* 2nd ed. Philadelphia: Saunders, 2001.
23. Young J: A closer look at I.V. fluids. *Nursing* 28:52–55, 1998.
24. Hand H: The use of intravenous therapy. *Nurs Standard* 15:47–55, 2001.
25. American Thoracic Society: Evidence-based colloid use in the critically ill: American Thoracic Society consensus statement. *Am J Respir Crit Care Med* 170:1247–1259, 2004.
26. Talecris Biotherapeutics: Plasma Protein Fraction (Human) 5%, USP, Plasmanate. Research Triangle Park, NC: Talecris Biotherapeutics, Inc., 2005, www.talecris-pi.info/insert/Plasmanate.pdf; accessed on January 20, 2007.
27. Talecris Biotherapeutics: Albumin (Human) 5%, USP, Plasmabumin-5. Research Triangle Park, NC: Talecris Biotherapeutics, Inc., 2005, www.talecris-pir.info/insert/Plasbumin25.pdf; accessed on January 20, 2007.
28. B Braun: HESpan. Irvine, CA: B Braun Medical, Inc., 2003, www.fda.gov/cder/foi/label/2003/BN890105s15lbl.pdf; accessed on January 20, 2007.

29. Gaspard KJ: Hematopoietic systems. In Porth CM (ed.): *Pathophysiology: Concepts of Altered Health States,* 7th ed. Philadelphia: Lippincott Williams & Wilkins, 2005.

30. Gaspard KJ: Disorders of hemostatsis. In Porth CM (ed.): *Pathophysiology: Concepts of Altered Health States,* 7th ed. Philadelphia: Lippincott Williams & Wilkins, 2005.

31. Rudnicke C: Transfusion alternatives. *J Infus Nurs* 26:29–33, 2003.

32. Blajchman MA, Vamvakas EC: Focus on research: The continuing risk of transfusion-transmitted infections. *N Engl J Med* 355:1303–1305, 2006.

33. Corwin HL, Carson JL: Blood transfusions: When is more really less? *N Engl J Med* 356:1667–1669, 2007.

34. Raghavan M, Marik PE: Anemia, allogenic blood transfusion, and immunomodulation in the critically ill. *Chest* 127:295–307, 2005.

35. Weir JA: Blood component therapy. In Hankins J, Lonsway RAW, Hedrick C, Perdue MB (eds.): *The Infusion Nurses Society: Infusion Therapy in Clinical Practice,* 2nd ed. Philadelphia: Saunders, 2001.

36. Miller R: Blood component therapy. *Urol Nurs* 22:331–339, 2002.

37. Richards NM, Giuliano KK: Transfusion practices in critical care: Essential care before and after a blood transfusion. *Am J Nurs* 102:S16–S22, 2002.

38. Fitzpatrick L: When to administer modified blood products. *Nursing* 32:36–41, 2002.

39. Osby MA, Saxena S, Nelson J, Shulman I: Safe handling and administration of blood components: Review of practical concepts. *Arch Pathol Lab Med* 131:690–694, 2007.

40. Tovarelli T, Valenti J: The pregnant Jehovah's Witness: How nurse executives can assist staff in providing culturally competent care. *JONA's Healthcare Law Ethics Regul* 7:105–109, 2005.

41. NWS Enteral/Parenteral Nutrition Interest Group: Continuing education. *Parenteral nutrition support* 63:54–57, 2006.

42. Wilson JM, Jordan JL: Parenteral nutrition. In Hankins J, Lonsway RAW, Hedrick C, Perdue MB (eds.): *The Infusion Nurses Society: Infusion Therapy in Clinical Practice,* 2nd ed. Philadelphia: Saunders, 2001.

43. Worthington P, Gilbert KA, Wagner BA: Parenteral nutrition for the acutely ill. *AACN Clin Issues* 11:559–579, 634–636, 2000.

44. Mirtello JM: Complications associated with drug and nutrient interactions. *J Infus Nurs* 27:19–24, 2004.

45. Hadaway LC: Administering parenteral nutrition with other I.V. drugs. *Nursing* 25:26, 2005.

46. Brogden BJ: Current practice in administration of parenteral nutrition: Venous access. *Br J Nurs* 13:1068–1073, 2004.

47. Lyman B: Metabolic complications associated with parenteral nutrition. *J Infus Nurs* 25:36–44, 2002.

48. Btaiche IF, Khalid N: Metabolic complications of parenteral nutrition in adults, part 1. *Am J Health Syst Pharm* 61:1938–1949, 2004.

49. Douglas JB, Hedrick C: Pharmacology. In Hankins J, Lonsway RAW, Hedrick C, Perdue MB (eds.): *The Infusion Nurses Society: Infusion Therapy in Clinical Practice,* 2nd ed. Philadelphia: Saunders, 2001.

50. Foster L, Wallis M, Peterson B, James H: A descriptive study of peripheral intravenous catheters in patients admitted to a pediatric unit in one Australian hospital. *J Infus Nurs* 25:159–167, 2002.

51. Spandorfer PR, Alessandrini EA, Joffe MD, et al.: Oral versus intravenous rehydration of moderately dehydrated children: A randomized, controlled trial. *Pediatrics* 115:295–301, 2005.

52. Frey AM: Intravenous therapy in children. In Hankins J, Lonsway RAW, Hedrick C, Perdue MB (eds.): *The Infusion Nurses Society: Infusion Therapy in Clinical Practice,* 2nd ed. Philadelphia: Saunders, 2001.

53. Gordon B, Crips J, Nagy S, et al.: Children's efforts to make sense of intravenous cannulation. *Austral Nurs J* 10:1–3, 1993.

54. Knue M, Doellman D, Jacobs BR: Peripherally inserted central catheters in children. *J Infus Nurs* 29:28–33, 2006.

55. Tan LH, Hess B, Diaz LK, et al.: Survey of the use of peripherally inserted central venous catheters in neonates with critical congenital cardiac disease. *Cardiol Young* 17:196–201, 2007.

56. Knue M, Doellman D, Rabin K, Jacobs BR: The efficacy and safety of blood sampling through peripherally inserted central catheter devices in children. *J Infus Nurs* 28:30–35, 2005.

57. Walther K: Intravenous therapy in the older adult. In Hankins J, Lonsway RAW, Hedrick C, Perdue MB (eds.): *The Infusion Nurses Society: Infusion Therapy in Clinical Practice,* 2nd ed. Philadelphia: Saunders, 2001.

58. Stechmiller JK: Early nutritional screening of older adults. *J Infus Nurs* 26:170–177, 2003.

59. Fetter MS: Geriatric assessment and management protocols: Issues for home infusion therapy providers. *J Infus Nurs* 26:153–160, 2003.

60. Zwicker CD: The elderly patient at risk. *J Infus Nurs* 26:137–143, 2003.

61. Mion LC, O'Connell A: Parenteral hydration and nutrition in the geriatric patient. *J Infus Nurs* 26:144–152, 2003.

62. Horgas AL: Pain management in elderly adults. *J Infus Nurs* 26:161–165, 2003.

63. Patel RB: Polypharmacy and the elderly. *J Infus Nurs* 26:166–169, 2003.

64. Mordock N: Intravenous therapy in the alternative care setting. In Hankins J, Lonsway RAW, Hedrick C, Perdue MB (eds.): *The Infusion Nurses Society: Infusion Therapy in Clinical Practice,* 2nd ed. Philadelphia: Saunders, 2001.

65. Lonsway RA: Intravenous therapy in the home. In Hankins J, Lonsway RAW, Hedrick C, Perdue MB (eds.): *The Infusion Nurses Society: Infusion Therapy in Clinical Practice,* 2nd ed. Philadelphia: Saunders, 2001.

INDEX

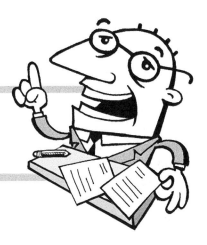

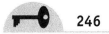

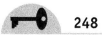